LEADERS
IN
RESPIRATORY ORGANS

BY

E. B. NASH, MD

NEW CENTRAL BOOK AGENCY

INDIA

First Published 1909
First NCBA Edition 2007

Publisher
NEW CENTRAL BOOK AGENCY (P) LTD
8/1 Chintamoni Das Lane, Kolkata 700 009

Distribution & Marketing
NEW CENTRAL BOOK AGENCY (P) LTD
8/1 Chintamoni Das Lane, Kolkata 700 009

Printing
NEW CENTRAL BOOK AGENCY (P) LTD
[Web-Offset Division]
Dhulagori, Sankrail, Howrah

Cover Design
Soumen Paul

ISBN 81-7381-533-X

Price: **Rs 95.00** (Rupees Ninety-five only)

DEDICATED TO

THE BRITISH HOMOEOPATHIC ASSOCIATION WHO ENTERTAINED ME SO ROYALLY WHILE WITH THEM. IT WAS A GREAT PLEASURE TO ME.

TABLE OF CONTENTS

PREFACE

The object of this unpretentious work is to place before the busy practitioner the indications, especially the *leading* ones, in a different way from that usually found in the ordinary textbooks. To the beginner, arranging the remedies in alphabetical order, without regard to the different stages of diseases, is rather confusing. It may justly be claimed that this way of mine has a tendency to lead to routinism. I have tried to guard against that by repeatedly assuring my readers that *any remedy* might be indicated in *any stage* of a complaint, and if so they must not be ignored. As will be seen, I have purposely avoided taking up time and space with the pathology and diagnosis of disease as found in the textbooks, my reasons being that, important as that may be, after all the selection of the remedy according to our art, according to symptomological indications, is of far more importance for CURATIVE PURPOSES. By this method of *symptom-covering* we are enabled to cure many a disease which cannot with certainty be named, and about which the best diagnosticians living would widely differ. I hope I will not be misunderstood, and be thought to place too low and estimate upon *diagnosis* and *pathology,* but rather as one who has tested the value of *Similia Similibus Curantur* from the standpoint of Hahnemann's clear teachings and is willing still to *stand for it.*

On account of a busy practice, college duties, etc., I have not been able to do so much as I could wish along this line. But my books so far have received so warm a welcome at home and abroad that I hope that this one more may be considered favourably, and not a *perpetration.*

I have had valuable help in the preparation of the condensed repertory at the end of the work, who modestly prefer not to have their names mentioned.

DR E. B. NASH

Port Dickinson, N.Y.

LEADERS IN

RESPIRATORY ORGANS

CATARRH.

ACUTE NASAL CATARRH.

(a) *Causes*—An acute coryza or Rhinitis may be an initial symptom of an *infection* like *influenza* or *measles;* more commonly it is primary—a "cold in the head." Its epidemic and contagious character is so marked that it probably depends upon germ infection. The chief predisposing causes are exposure to cold, variable weather and inhalation of irritating vapors.

(b) *Symptoms.*—There is chilliness, headache, slight fever (100° to 101°) and sneezing, with quickened pulse, dry skin and throat. Some backache and general aching are not uncommon. The nasal mucous membrane swells, so that "mouth-breathing" is imperative, and there is a thin acrid discharge from the nostrils. The eyes water, the senses of taste and smell are impaired, the pharynx is reddened, the throat is sore and the neck stiff, and slight dysphagia may be present. Herpes of the nose and lips is common. The larynx may be involved, causing hoarseness; the trachea and bronchi, cough; the Eustachian tubes, slight deafness.

In a day or two the nasal discharge increases, becomes thicker and muco-purulent, and in 5 or 6 days the swelling of the mucosa and associated symptoms subside. The coryzal discharge persists for a week or two longer.

(c) *Diagnosis.*—Ordinarily easy, but the possibility that it is the initial coryza of measles or influenza is to be borne in mind. (Butler).

This is perhaps as good a condensed desciiption of Acute Nasal Catarrh as could be given, but the question as to the possibility or probability of germ infection ought to be settled, in order to enable the proper hound (germicide) to be set on the track of the germ. Another thing deserves passing notice before we enter into the therapeutics of this affection, *i. e.*, the discharge is not always acrid as Butler states. It may be acrid or bland. It may be acrid from the nose and non-irritating from the eyes or *vice versa.* Other finer points necessary to be observed by the homœopathic prescriber will be mentioned as we go through the indications for the remedies.

THERAPEUTICS.

If the primary cause is the "cold in the head" from exposure simply, and not of the epidemic variety, it is important to known what *kind* of exposure it was.

Aconite. Is adapted to such suffering from exposure to *dry cold air.* Chill or coldness followed by fever heat and restlessness, headache at the root of the nose, not much coryza as yet; or habitual coryza suppressed; *burning and pricking in the throat and Eustachian tubes* are symptoms commonly found indicating this remedy. If given early in frequent doses for an hour or two the fever will abate and be followed by perspiration and general relief of all the symptoms.

There is another remedy not so often used as it ought to be, and it comes before the reaction from the chilly stage has occurred, which calls for *Aconite*, viz:—

Camphor. *Icy cold;* cold *subjectively* and *objectively.* The blood seems to have receded from the surface, especially the extremities. It is like the collapse of cholera. The nose is stopped, dry, and pointed. The head aches in the frontal sinuses, even throbs.

Now seat yourself by the fire, and take a drop on sugar, every five minutes, of common spirits of *Camphor* until reaction sets in, and there is an end of that cold. It is especially efficacious after a ride in the cold air, until thoroughly chilled through, even prostrated by the cold.

Anyone who understands the principles of Homœopathy can see how *Camphor* is here the remedy. But it is in the very first stage of a cold that it is to be used. After reaction sets in *Aconite* or some other remedy will be indicated.

Nux vomica is another splendid remedy for the first stage of a "cold." The nose is stopped, or *stops at night and runs through the day.* There is *frontal headache.* Throat sore and very sensitive to *inhaled cold air*. But the most characteristic indication is that the patient is *chilly on the least motion or uncovering*. *Even during the fever*, must be covered and keep quiet.

These three remedies, according to indications as above, will often serve to check a cold and prevent the fluent coryza, or fluent stage which will follow in the general course of the disease, if left to itself.

Bryonia may follow *Aconite* or *Nux vom.*, if notwithstanding these remedies the nose remains dry and obstructed, and the headache over the *root of the nose* persists and is greatly *aggravated on motion.* The lips are parched and dry, and there is much thirst. If the first stage is passed and the fluent coryza has set in another class of remedies comes in, such as—

Mercurius. With this remedy there are *creeping chills;* worse in the evening and night, even in bed. The nose discharges thin water with sneezing and lachrymation and sore throat, which *stings* and *pricks*, with a cons ant inclination to swallow saliva which accumulates in abundance, accompanied with a bad smell from the mouth. There may be fever and later on *profuse sweat, which however does not relieve.*

Allium cepa may dispute place with *Mercurius*, so far as fluent coryza and lachrymation are concerned. The discharge from the nose is *profuse, watery and corrosive.* It *corrodes the nose and upper lip*, and is worse in the evening and in doors, and *better in open air.* It has also profuse lachrymation, with burning, biting and smarting in the eyes, but the discharge unlike that from the nose is *bland.* It does not excoriate the cheeks as does the nasal discharge the nose and upper lip (*Euphrasia* is exactly the reverse, *i. e.*, corrosive lachrymation and bland nasal discharge). There may be headache and that is also worse in warm room and *better in open air.* This remedy is particularly useful in children, when the profuse coryza or cold extends downward to the bronchi, with a like *profuse secretion in the tubes, with cough and much rattling of mucus.*

Arsenicum follows well either of these three remedies (*Merc.*, *Euph.* and *Cepa*) in fluent coryza, when neither of them seem sufficient, but the discharge becomes more BURNING in character. The throat also *burns* but is relieved by *hot drinks* so long as they are running over the part. The chill and heat alternate or intermingle. There is generally amelioration from *heat* of room, or hot local applications. There is also greater weakness and prostration than with the other remedies and the whole case is aggravated at night; *especially at midnight.*

Four more remedies that might be used oftener than they are—*Sabadilla*, *Arum tri.*, *Sang. nit.*, and *Kali iod.*

Sabadilla. Has profuse sneezing and lachrymation which is decidedly aggravated in open air and *bright light.* There is often sore throat running from left to right like *Lachesis*, but unlike it there is desire for *hot drinks*, which ameliorate. There is also a sensation as of a lump in the throat which creates *constant necessity to swallow.*

It is especially useful in hay-fever or hay-fever subjects. Every time he takes cold it settles in his nose and throat.

Arum triphyllum is an excessive irritant to the nose, mouth and throat. The discharge is ichorous, and the *surfaces raw red and sometimes bloody*, with a sensation which causes the patient to bore with his fingers into the sensitive and raw surfaces. There is also sore throat and hoarseness with continually *changing or breaking voice.*

Sanguinaria nitrate irritates intensely the nose, eyes, throat and bronchi. The throat is dry and burns, as does also the nose. This sensation of rawness and burning extends all through the nose, posterior nares and throat. The third and sixth trituration of this remedy dry on the tongue once in two or three hours will sometimes check the progress of such a cold and prevent its running through all its stages.

Further use of the remedy will serve to draw out more positive characteristics so that it can be used higher.

Kali iodatum. Redness and swelling of the nose, with constant discharge of watery, acrid, colorless liquid.

Œdematous swelling of the eyelids with lachrymation. It is especially to be used after *Mercury* has done all it can, or fails; and more especially in syphilitic subjects who have been abused by *Mercury*. Such subjects are liable to repeated violent attacks of acrid coryza with bloated eyelids.

The above remedies are, according to indications,

able to cure ordinary "colds" or coryzas and the consequences of them, if skillfully applied.

If after these two stages are passed anything more is needed we have

Pulsatilla, which is generally the best remedy if there is *that bland discharge* from the nose, or the same kind of expectoration with the cough. The sense of smell is blunted or *lost*, also *taste*, or *bitter* taste. There is no thirst, and generally poor appetite. The choice may lie between this remedy and

Mercurius solubilis, but *Mercurius* is weak and *sweats* easily, or at night in bed, and the mouth is moist, with bad smell, flabby tongue with indented edges, and *thirst*.

Sulphur follows well either of these two remedies, especially in psoric constitutions, and will often "finish up" the case and prevent its running into the chronic form.

We said, of the *diagnosis* of this disease, that it was "ordinarily easy, but the possibility that it is the initial coryza of measles or influenza is to be borne in mind."

If it is measles we will bear in mind such remedies as *Aconite*, *Gelsemium*, *Euphrasia*, and *Pulsatilla*. That does not come within the scope of this work. But

INFLUENZA

or, as it is now popularly known, *La Grippe* we will have to notice.

What distinguishes influenza (which is really nothing more than a violent catarrhal fever) from other fevers of this class is the circumstance, that influenza attacks the whole nervous system at once. Sometimes with rheumatic pains in the limbs. More or less lameness, fever; and inflammatory symptoms which may increase to a genuine acute bronchitis or pleuritis. This disease which for a few years seemed to be modified in intensity from what it was when it first broke out in Europe (fifty years ago) has seemed to revive its former severity in the last ten or fifteen years, so that many cases are utterly prostrated by it, and long lasting effects follow.

One of the best and oftenest indicated remedies is the one discovered by accident when this malady was at its beginning so severe and general, and the symptoms so uniform that it was "dubbed" "*break-bone-fever*," and the remedy, on account of its efficacy called "*bone-set*," is

Eupatorium perfoliatum. Deep seated, aching all over as if in the bones, especially severe in the *back*, *wrists* and *ankles*. There is also severe bruised *soreness* (*Arnica*) so that the patient is worse on motion (*Bryon.*) (although he feels very restless (*Rhus*)) even to the muscles of the eyes as expressed in the symptom—"*eyeballs sore on turning them*," watery coryza often present, but may be absent, also nausea, or vomiting and prostration. The choice often lies between this remedy, in the first stage of the disease, and

Gelsemium. With this remedy the *general prostration* is very marked; wants to lie perfectly still, and *trembles* from weakness from the least exertion;

even the hands tremble when lifting them up; the eyelids droop from weakness. It seems almost a semi-paralytic state. There is fever, but little or no thirst, the tongue *trembles* when protruding it. The sensorium is in accord with the general weakness; *blunted*, but little or no dilirium.

Bryonia alba stands about midway between *Eupatorium* and *Gelsemium.* Like them it is better when quiet and greatly aggravated on *motion*, the face turns pale on rising and he faints or is *nauseated* and *stitching* pain in various parts are prominent. It must come early into the case if there are the stitching pains in the pleura. All three remedies have *aching pains*, but *Eupatorium* is "bone pains." *Gelsemium* muscular or myalgia. *Bryonia* intermixed with *stitching* pains. One or the other of these three remedies will in the majority of cases, according to my observation, control the case, or so modify it as to make the subsequent treatment easy.* But if they should not; such remedies as *Causticum*, *Rhus tox.*, *Arsenicum*, *Sulphur*, etc., will be necessary to finish the case. Either one

---

*Dr. Clarke, of London, finds *Baptisia* the nearest specific. This is very high authority and must not be ignored. It certainly has many symptoms in common with this disease. Another remedy which he mentioned is *Phytolacca* when the throat is inflamed and spotty like tonsillitis (follicular) and I have often verified his statement in such cases, and when we remember that the aching, soreness and fever of la grippe and tonsillitis it would be no very remarkable mistake to confound the two complaints in the beginning. The *Natrum salycilic* also spoken of by him I have never yet tried, but the *Kali iod.* and *Psorinum* are fine, for the weakness during convalescence, the *Kali iod.*, especially according to indications as given under bronchitis.

of the above described forms of catarrhal inflammation, may, on account of complications, or of our being called in too late to apply our treatment in time, run into laryngitis, bronchitis, pneumonia, etc. Then we will be obliged to treat them according to our art, as will be described when treating these affections. But without involving these organs to any great degree, we may have following as the result of recurring attacks of the acute form:

CHRONIC NASAL CATARRH.

It may also be caused by syphilis and tuberculosis. It may appear in three forms. *Simple Chronic Catarrh*—in which the mucous membrane becomes congested and swollen, sometimes to the degree of *stenosis.* It may be dry or with an abundant thick secretion. All this may occur repeatedly on "catching cold," to which the patient is *very liable.* If this persists the "lower turbinals are swollen and enlarged, there is constant hawking to remove the thick secretion from the upper pharynx, and the patient becomes a 'mouth-breather' to a varying extent. In the majority of cases the pharyngeal mucosa and adenoid tissues are coincidently affected, constituting a chronic naso-pharyngeal catarrh. The voice becomes nasal, and varying degrees of deafness are common." Post nasal dropping is also common. It is then called *Hypertrophic Rhinitis.* Another form of chronic catarrh, called *Atrophic Rhinitis*, "may be, but is by no means necessarily, a sequence of the *hypertrophic* form. The horrible and disgusting odor (*ozæna*) which is the principle symptom of the disease, is met with also as an evidence of syphilis, disease of the nasal bones, glanders, and foreign bodies. The sense of smell is abolished. On inspection, the nasal mucosa is seen to be shrunken and atrophied, with a resultant unusual roominess of the nasal chambers. The thick purulent secretion coating the membrane, dries into yellowish-green adherent crusts, which emit the offensive odour."

So far as this classification is concerned, it is not possible to draw a line of demarkation so distinct that it would invaribly indicate where recurrent acute catarrh left off and the chronic form began; and so far as the treatment is concerned, the symptoms would have to decide the choice of remedies whether the disease be one of the recurrent acute form or the chronic form flaming up so as to simulate it.

Lycopodium is one of the best remedies if the catarrh is of the dry form; *stoppage of the nose at night*, so that the patient has to breathe through the mouth. If given not lower than the 30th and not too frequently and at too short intervals, it will cure many cases and prevent adenoids, or remove by curing them. Of course the other *Lycopodium* symptoms and constitution will in greater or less degree be found present.

Hepar sulphur. If the patient's nose stuffs up tight on *any exposure to the cold air;* and is extremely sensitive to cold air, which brings on the catarrh, croup or cough. It is especially useful in cases that have taken *Mercury* in large doses.

Sticta pulmonaria is not only useful in acute colds, where there is severe pain in the forehead and root of the nose before the discharge sets in, but in the chronic form it is just as good. The nose is stuffed up with the same pressure and fullness in the root of the nose and frontal sinuses, and the nasal secretion dries up and sticks, causing a constant desire to blow the nose, or forms into scabs difficult to dislodge. In some cases mucus drops from the posterior nares, and the throat looks raw and feels like dried leather. Sometimes the choice will lie between this remedy and

Kali bichromicum, which also has many scabs or "clinkers," and similar pains over the root of the nose, especially when the discharge becomes suppre sed by cold or other causes. It also has a post nasal discharge, and it is apt to be tough and ropy like all the mucous discharges of this remedy. Then again *Kali bich.* takes a deeper hold upon the tissues than *Sticta*. The nostrils fill with dry hard crusts, that are often bloody when discharged. The septum ulcerates or round ulcers penetrate, or sometimes entirely destroy it. This state of things may occur with or without a syphilitic element in the case. In syphilitic cases of course there is offensive smell attending such deep seated disorganizations. In syphilitic ozæna—

Kali iodatum may be preferable, especially in those cases that have been abused by *Mercury*. In such cases we may have repeated attacks of apparently acute coryza, but otherwise there may be accumulations of very tenacious mucus in the nostrils, or discharges of *greenish black*, cr yellow matter smelling foul, or like the *Kali bich.* may have ulcerations, but they involve the frontal sinuses and antrum rather than the septum. The remedy that forms a valuable trio with *Kali bich.* and *iod.* is—

Aurum; in the form of the metal or muriate. It eats more deeply than either of them, involving the bones of the nose. Leading Symptoms—Crusts in the nose; obstructed, ulcerated, agglutinated, painful nostrils, ozæna; thick fetid discharge, severe frontal headache, *caries.* The patient is melancholy even to suicide. Like the Kali's it is especially useful in cases that have been abused by *Mercury* or *Kali iod.* or both. Two remedies that occur to me with the last three, and which perhaps ought to have preceded them here as they generally do in the course of a chronic catarrh, are

Pulsatilla and *Kali sulphuricum.* The former is first to be considered in a chronic catarrh, which has followed one or several acute attacks. The thin watery discharge of the first stage has changed to thick green, bland, sometimes offensive, with loss of taste and smell. The nasal mucus becomes offensive as of old catarrh, it is worse in the *evening* and in a *warm room*, as is the patient generally, or, in other words, it is *better in the open air.* The—

Kali sulphuricum is so like the *Pulsatilla* that it deserves the name of its "chronic," and if *Pulsatilla* does not cure such a case, and it tends to get worse instead of better, *Kali sul.* will complement it very nicely. This is so, not only in catarrh of the nose, but also where the process continues downward to bronchi and lungs. It is especially useful where there is much rattling of mucus remaining. Of course—

Sulphur and *Calcarea ostrearum* will never be forgotten in chronic diseases of any kind. Both have the chronic form of catarrh, with thick, fetid, purulent discharge of offensive smell, etc., *Sulphur* suiting the psoric constitution and temperament, and *Calcarea* the leucophlegmatic. Indeed the choice of such remedies will often rest on general indications rather than the local. In fact, these must also enter into all prescriptions of *any remedy*, no matter how strong the local indications. *The whole patient must be considered.*

Our list of remedies might be extended to much greater length, and indeed the whole materia medica or any of the remedies so far mentioned or not mentioned may be called into requisition in all forms of nasal catarrh. And here again we desire to emphasize, lest we be misunderstood, that we, as homœopaths, do not treat local manifestations to the exclusion of the other abnormal symptoms which characterize the sickness of the patient. But some remedies do act by preference on certain localities and organs, and when the so-called disease manifests the same kind of preference, or centers its force in such localities, the remedy having both the general and local manifestations in its pathogenesis is the one to use.

We will now mention in alphabetical order some more remedies with indications that have been found reliable when coupled with the general indications which must correspond.

Æsculus hippocastanum. Fluent coryza, dull frontal headache, thin, watery discharge, burning, rawness, sensitive to inhaled air (*Nux v.*).

Ailanthus glandulosa. Copious, thin, ichorous and bloody discharge from the nose (Scarlatina).

Ammonium carbonicum. Nose stopped at night; mouth breathing.

Asafœtida. Discharge of very offensive matter from the nose; with caries of the bone.

Corrallium rubrum. Profuse secretion of mucus dropping into posterior nares, obliging frequent hawking; inspired air feels cold.

Dulcamara. Dry coryza, stoppage of nose, or coryza suppressed, or < from least exposure to damp cold air.

Graphites. Chronic nasal catarrh; internal nose dry, with dry scabs with sore, cracked and crusty nostrils (*Ant. crud.*). Sore on blowing it.

Hydrastis Can. Stuffiness of nares, discharge of thick, yellow and stringy mucus, or dropping down into posterior nares. So profuse as to be raised in long tenacious strings (*Kali bich.*). Ozæna with purulent, bloody discharge.

Kali mur. Catarrh extending to the Eustachian tubes.

Lachesis. Complaints from suppressed catarrh; > by the restoration of discharge.

Natrum muriaticum. Acute coryza with clear, profuse, watery, white discharge, like in hay fever; or chronic catarrh with sore wings and scabs in the nose.

Natrum sulphuricum. Chronic catarrh, both ante and post nasal, discharge yellow or green < in *damp weather*.

Nitricum acidum. Discharge acrid, watery, offensive, corroding upper lip in scarlatina, diphtheria or syphilis; or cracks, or ulcerations of nostrils, scurfy, bloody matter, with *pricking as from splinters in the nose.*

Petroleum. Ozæna, scabs and purulent mucus, nose sore, nostrils cracked, extending to Eustachian tube.

Phosphorus. Frequent blowing of blood from the nose; handkerchief is always bloody, chronic catarrh.

Psorinum. Is, like *Sulphur*, always to be carefully considered in psoric subjects. This is like *Hepar*, *Sulphur*, *Silicea* and *Tuberculinum*, very susceptible to cold air or change of weather, wants to wear a fur cap, overcoat or shawl even in the hottest weather. It is also especially useful in chronic catarrh with purulent or bloody discharge which may be yellowish-green, like the expectoration. It is dropping from posterior nares so as to awaken at night. Hawking of lumpy mucus gives temporary relief.

Sambucus. Nose stopped up tight, especially in children "snuffles."

Sepia. Dry coryza, nostrils sore, ulcerated, scabby, discharge large, green, offensive smelling plugs.

Silicea. Chronic coryza, ulcers high up in the nose, fetid, offensive discharges, caries of bones, from syphilis or scrofula. > *from having head wrapped up warm.*

Thuja occidentalis. Much thick, green mucus with blood and pus; brown scabs form, which are painful, sycotic diathesis.

Tuberculinum must not be forgotten when the patient is continually "taking cold," says the least exposure brings on a new cold. This is especially to be regarded if the patient has a tuberculous history. It is often the beginning of consumption, and may be checked by this remedy, if given high and at not too frequent intervals.

REPERTORY TO NASAL SYMPTOMS.

We will conclude this part of our subject by giving a few remedies in a sort of repertorial form, as leaders to a fuller study of them. I have purposely not allowed more than seven to come under one list, because it would not be advisable to do so. I have also meant to arrange them as far as I could in the order of their importance.

DRY CORYZA (no discharge).—*Nux vomica*, *Sticta*, *Lycopodium*, *Camphor*, *Ammonium carb.*, *Sambucus*, *Bryonia.*

NOSTRILS OBSTRUCTED.—*Nux vomica*, *Sticta*, *Ammonium carb.*, *Lycopodium*, *Kali bichromicum*, *Pulsatilla*, *Sambucus.*

CORYZA FLUENT, OR THIN, WATERY DISCHARGE.—*Allium cepa*, *Mercurius*, *Arsenicum*, *Sabadilla*, *Euphrasia*, *Kali iodatum*, *Sanguinaria nitrate.*

DISCHARGE CORROSIVE OR EXCORIATING.—*Allium cepa*, *Arsenicum*, *Arum triphyl.*, *Nitric acid*, *Bromium*, *Sanguinaria nit.*

DISCHARGE BLAND.—*Pulsatilla*, *Euphrasia*, *Kali sulph.*

DISCHARGE GREEN.—*Pulsatilla*, *Mercurius*, *Sepia*, *Kali iodatum.*

DISCHARGE YELLOW.—*Pulsatilla*, *Kali sulph.*, *Kali bichrom.*, *Sepia*, *Sulphur*, *Lycopodium*, *Aurum.*

CRUSTS AND SCABS.—*Sticta*, *Kali bichrom.*, *Sepia*, *Thuja*, *Natrum arsenicatum*, *Aurum.*

OFFENSIVE.—*Aurum*, *Asafœtida*, *Pulsatilla*, *Mercurius*, *Hepar sulph.*

PURULENT.—*Mercurius*, *Hepar sulph.*, *Aurum*, *Kali bichrom.*, *Silicea.*

STRINGY DISCHARGE.—*Kali bichrom.*, *Hydrastis*, *Sanicula.*

DISCHARGE FROM POSTERIOR NARES.—*Corralium*, *Mercurius protoiod.*, *Ferrum*, *Cinnabaris*, *Hydrastis*, *Natrum carb.*, *Natrum mur.*, *Psorinum.*

HAY FEVER.—*Sabadilla*, *Allium cepa*, *Gelsemium*, *Lachesis*, *Sinapis nig.*, and *Mountain air*; WORSE IN THE MORNING, *Nux vomica*; < IN THE EVENING, *Allium cepa.*

OZÆNA.—*Aurum*, *Kali bichrom.*, *Mercurius*, *Pulsatilla*, *Sepia*, *Silicea*, *Hepar sulph.*

PAINS IN THE BONES OF THE NOSE.—*Aurum*, *Kali bichrom.*, *Kali iod.*

WORSE AT NIGHT.—*Mercurius*, *Aurum.*

PRESSING AT THE ROOT.—*Sticta*, *Kali bichrom.*, *Mercurius biniod.*, *Pulsatilla.*

SENSATION OF RAWNESS.—*Æsculus*, *Arum triphyl.*, *Mercurius corr.*, *Kali iodaıum.*

SORENESS INSIDE.—*Arum triphyl.*, *Æsculus*, *Kali bichrom.*, *Nitric acid*, *Silicea*, *Aurum.*

SMELL LOST.—*Pulsatilla*, *Hepar sulph.*, *Mercurius.*

SNEEZING. — *Allium cepa*, *Mercurius*, *Sabadilla*, *Arsenicum*, *Cyclamen*, *Carbo vegetabilis.*

SNUFFLES.—*Nux vomica*, *Sambucus*, *Lycopodium.*

ULCERS INSIDE. — *Kali bichrom.*, *Aurum*, *Nitric acid*, *Sepia*, *Silicea*, *Thuja.*

LARYNGITIS.

Butler (Diagnostics) classifies this as follows:

Acute Catarrhal Laryngitis.

Acute Laryngitis with spasm of the glottis (croup).

Chronic Laryngitis.

Œdema of the Larynx.

Tuberculous Laryngitis.

Syphilitic Laryngitis.

Tumours of the Larynx.

Laryngismus stridulus and paralysis of the Larynx.

It is not the object in this work to write out the diagnosis of each of these forms of Laryngeal trouble, for that may be found in the many good works already written, such as Butler, Bartlett and others. We have to do with the leading indications of the *remedies* found most useful in the treatment of them. In fact, after the diagnosis is clearly made the symptoms which correspond between the patient and the pathogenesis of the remedy will have to guide to the choice. This is true whether the case be one coming from colds or other causes of acute Laryngitis or whether it be one originating in, or being complicated, by Syphilis, Psora, Sycosis, Tuberculosis, etc. It is lamentably true that many diseases are caused or aggravated by the misuse of drugs, and this, too, must be taken into the account.

A remedy may be indicated in several forms, both acute or chronic, as, for instance, *Bichromate of Potash* or *Hepar sulphur.*, so in giving our leaders we will feel free, or not, to mention varieties, etc.

Not giving the remedies in alphabetical order, as is done in most works, we may well begin this list with *Aconite*, as it has a decided and positive action on the larynx. *Aconite* is often indicated in the acute form, brought on by exposure to *cold dry air*, most works say cold west winds, and that depends on whether you are living on the Atlantic shores or the Pacific. Cold dry air is better; chill or chilliness, followed with fever, with hot, dry skin, great restlessness, impatience and *fearful anxiety.* The child wakes up in the night with croupy cough and breathing; pain in the larynx and anxious suffocation. With this remedy most cases can, if taken early, be cured in a short time or so modified that other remedies easily finish up the case. This is of course in cases uncomplicated with specific Miasms.

Belladonna may follow, or be preferable at the first, if instead of the *fearfulness* and anxiety there should be just as high or even higher temperature, the skin seeming fairly to radiate heat, or impart a burning feeling to the hand that touches it; there is *drowsiness* with twitching; spasmodic or barking cough, pain in the larynx, dark red, turgid face, throbbing carotids; dilated or contracted pupils; sweat on *covered parts* (*Acon.* dry) all the disease or vascular excitement tending to the head. Delirium is common with this remedy, and it is especially indicated if there is *dry soreness* of the throat.

Arum triphyllum. In acute or chronic forms of the

disease where there is hoarseness or rawness (*Caust.*) of the throat; can't control the voice, *breaks when trying to talk or sing;* dry cough at first, later with expectoration or accumulation of mucus. Especially useful for opera singers or public speakers who lose their voice (*Rhus tox.*).

Allium cepa. Violent catarrhal laryngitis, especially if accompanied or preceded by the characteristic coryza of this remedy, pain in larynx when coughing, causing the patient to grasp the larynx when coughing, < on inspiring cool air and in the evening.

Causticum. Acute or chronic when there is sense of *rawness* or soreness in throat and larynx, sometimes extending down the trachea, with soreness on coughing even through the whole chest. There may be partial or complete loss of voice; the hoarseness is generally < in the morning (*Carbo veg.* evening). Sometimes involuntary escape of urine with the cough.

Drosera. Hoarseness with very *deep bass* voice. Much cough especially after midnight; especially if it becomes spasmodic like whooping cough. The cough, also like the voice, has a deep trumpet tone, something like that of *Verbascum*, but the latter goes lower down than the larynx.

Hepar sul. Croupy cough < in the morning. The patient is very sensitive to dry cold winds, which bring on repeated attacks, and the cough is aggravated even if exposure of the body or a hand to cold air takes place. Generally there is rattling of loose mucus, but little is expectorated. Even asthmatic wheezing may be present. *Hepar* is a valuable remedy in both the acute and chronic form of the disease.

Apis. If *Belladonna* fails where there is much redness, stinging or an œdematous condition of the throat, or submucous tissue of the larynx, suffocative cough and dyspnœa, feels as though every breath would be the last, < by lying down and warmth. Of course this is mostly in the acute form of the disease.

Phosphorus. Hoarseness; lining of vocal cords highly injected, cough < by talking, laughing, singing, *cold air* or *lying on left side;* tickling in the larynx and spasmodic cough, followed by dryness and burning in the throat.

Spongia. Acute form with burning and tickling in the larynx; swelling of larynx with sensation of a *plug* in the throat; great hoarseness with sawing respiration, especially in threatened laryngeal phthisis.

Iodine. Especially in brunettes, with constant tickling cough with pain in the larynx, ulceration, great emaciation and hunger. Glandular swelling or dwindling. The general symptoms will guide to its choice better than the local.

Kali bich. The expectoration of stringy mucus is the chief indication. It draws out in long strings hanging down to the floor. The cough is < mornings and often nearly strangles him.

Calcarea ost. is useful in the *chronic form.* The patient *is very hoarse*, sometimes can only speak in a whisper; also roughness or sense of *rawness* in the larynx, all < in the morning. Expectoration also in the morning and during the day, little or none at night, though the cough may be worse. The general symptoms of the remedy are present in abundance, and it is especially useful in the well known *Calcarea ost.* temperament.

Carbo vegetabilis is also well adapted to the chronic form, though it may come in early and prevent it, if there is *hoarseness* equal to *Calcarea* or *Causticum*, but is < *in the evening* or the damp air of evening. It is particularly well adapted to old or elderly people of low or reduced vitality. With both *Calcarea* and *Carbo veg.* there may be thick heavy expectoration.

Argentum met. is useful in hoarseness of professional singers. Total loss of voice at times, always < by speaking or singing. The cricoid cartilage is painful, painful to touch with sensation of foreign body; over the bifurcation of trachea a raw spot, and coughs up a gelatinous phlegm.

These fifteen remedies are leading ones for the treatment of affections of the larynx, but not by any means all of them. For instance, *Aurum*, *Mercury*, *Kali iod.* might, and must, come into consideration for syphilitic cases, as must *Sulphur* and the other antipsorics in psoric complications and causes.

So far as local treatment of this affection is concerned, the specialist may come in for his share of the work; but even here an understanding of the homœopathic therapeutics will enable him to do infinitely better work than his allopathic neighbor who depends almost altogether on local measures. These local affections are almost always caused or complicated by constitutional states, and to ignore this is to miss the "main chance" for the best and most lasting benefit. Too many of our own men are drifting away from our superior therapeutics to the local treatment side of these affections.

The inevitable result of this is to cripple them, do injustice to those who have a right to expect better things of them than from the allopaths, and dishonor the name which they bear as subscribers to the doctrines of Hahnemann. The only advantage to arise from these departures is that they will not *cure* their patients, but, by deceiving them with palliations instead, may expect them back again and again for a repetition of the same treatment. Of course, there is *money* in that. If any man will practice medicine, either general or special, with the idea of money-making as his chief object, it seems to me that he is not entitled to the respect of God, man or the devil. It is to be hoped that there are few such on earth, and there'll never be one in heaven. One other thing I wish to mention in closing, local treatment alone is oftener merely suppression than cure, and this being the case the affection is very apt to locate where it cannot be reached by local measures, as, for instance, in the bronchi, lungs or elsewhere, and the "last state of that man is worse than the first." This is a most important truth and should not be ignored. If the laity only knew this they would shun doctors as a menace rather than resort to them for relief or cure.

CROUP.

As to the unanimity of the old school authorities in regard to this disease we may judge something by the following: "Membranous croup is in the large majority of cases laryngeal diphtheria; in a *small minority* (italics ours) streptococcus inflammation. It is usually secondary by extension from the pharynx, *occasionally* primary. A croupy cough, hoarseness or aphonia, and above all the evidences of progressive laryngeal stenosis, constitute the leading symptoms. As the narrowing of the glottic opening proceeds the breathing becomes stridulous and dyspnœa and cyanosis become manifest. The supraclavicular, episternal, intercostal, and epigastric spaces are deeply retracted with inspiration and bulge with expiration. The child is excessively restless, the nostrils are worked violently, and the sterno-mastoids become prominent during inspiration. Shreds of membrane may be coughed up. If the stenosis is not relieved the child passes into a semi-comatose state and finally dies. The fever is usually slight and the general condition of the patient good. The membrane may extend into the trachea and the bronchial tubes." (Butler).

"LARYNGEAL DIPHTHERIA."—*Membranous croup.*—With a very large proportion of all the cases of membranous laryngitis the Klebs-Loeffler bacillus is associated; in a much smaller number other organisms, particularly the streptococcus, are found. Membranous croup then may be said to be either genuine diphtheria or diphtheroid in character. Of 286 cases which the disease was confined to the larynx or bronchi, in 229 the Klebs-Loeffler bacilli were found. In 57 they were not present, but 17 of these cultures were unsatisfactory. (Park and Beebe).

The streptococcus cases are more likely to be secondary to other acute diseases. (Hare).

It will be noticed by these two authorities that two kinds of croup are recognized, the membranous and spasmodic, and that the presence of Klebs-Loeffler bacillus is not always present in true cases of the disease. Osler recognizes only one form of true croup. The spasmodic form is called "false croup." Mackenzie used to claim that the acute catarrhal form and the membranous variety were only different degrees of the same affection.

Our own Raue writes (special pathology): "True croup is most readily confounded with CATARRHAL LARYNGITIS or PSEUDO-CROUP; the latter, however, is frequently attended with other catarrhal symptoms, such as sneezing, coryza, etc., and is apt to occur frequently.

DIPHTHERIA is thought by some writers (Wagner and others) not to be an essentially different affection from croup, and that there is no sharp dividing line between the two. But if we take into consideration that in croup the exudation takes place *upon* the free surface of the mucous membrane, and in diphtheria also *within* it, causing necrosis and loss of substance, that diphtheria is contagious while croup is not, and that in many cases of diphtheria a peculiar penetrating smell from the mouth claims at once our attention, we shall hardly find any difficulty in distinguishing between the two, notwithstanding the close similarity of symptoms between them. This last was written before bacteriology took high rank as a means of diagnosis, and I am of the opinion with Rosenbach (see "Physician versus Bacteriologist") and others that the presence or absence of the microbe for purposes of diagnosis is not all there is of it. While we would not underestimate the value of bacteriology as a biological science, the importance of the study of the microscopical world, and should be well aware of the surprising biological information, and important methods found in the study of bacteriology, we are convinced that all the claims of the *nothing but bacteriologists* cannot be allowed. These diagnosticians *in absentia* need not expect us, who are at the bedside taking into account the *whole case*, to stand aside upon their *ipse dixit*.

Again while it is important for several reasons that we should be able, if possible to say whether a case is diphtheritic or not, it is equally, and, I think, more important to select the similimum in the treatment of the case, especially as that similimum must be used in some stage of both diseases. For instance, *Kali bichromicum*, *Hepar sulph.* and the *Iodine* may be indicated in either croup or diphtheria, according to indications. So in our *leading* indications for remedies we will cover (or try to) the ground for *croup*, whether catarrhal or diphtheritic.

Aconite will relieve nine-tenths of the cases of catarrhal laryngitis or croup as it occurs in our northern latitudes. It generally occurs as the result of exposure to *dry, cold air*, attacking the child in the evening or first part of the night, with great excitement, high fever, tossing and gasping for breath. A little of the 12th or 30th dilution in water in teaspoonful doses once in ten or 15 minutes, until the child becomes more quiet, and then at longer intervals until the fever subsides, will be all that is necessary if administered early in the disease. If, however, the cough persists with a rough, croupy sound, as of a "saw driven through a pine board," and the stridulous breathing continues between the paroxysms *Spongia* is apt to be the next remedy. If the cough becomes more rattling, but still croupy, as if the mucus would come up but does not, and the aggravations are in the latter part of the night or morning, and especially if all the symptoms are made worse by cold air striking the patient, *Hepar sulphur.* comes in. These three were Bœnninghausen's great remedies, and with them he had success never before his time attained. He gave them in the 200th. They are still as useful as then, and must always be, because Homœopathy is always the same. But there are cases that will not respond to this treatment, which proves that routinism won't do.

Iodine is a wonderful remedy in croup if occurring in dark complexioned, black eyed children. The child grasps at its throat during the paroxysm, and cries as if in pain; the fever and restlessness are almost equal to *Aconite*. It follows well after *Hepar*.

Bromine follows well after *Spongia*, when the aggravation sets in the next evening, is best suited to light haired, light complexioned children; gasps for breath, wants to be carried, but very quickly, saying run, run; long-drawn-out inhalation, and great prostration. It is especially useful where the trouble seems to start low down in diphtheria.

Kali bichromicum is suited to all cases of the common croup or diphtheria, if the membranous deposit is positive, and there is ropy mucus discharged from the mouth and sometimes nose. I have had the pleasure of curing several bad cases of diphtheritic croup with this remedy.

Phosphorus is especially useful when the violence of the attack has been broken by some of the foregoing, but there remains a tendency to relapse; the child grows worse again every evening, or the cough goes down in the tubes and lungs. It will often clean up the case, in desperate cases where other remedies have failed in both forms of croup

Arsenicum may still avail. The child grows excessively restless, weak, and is especially worse at midnight. In one desperate case of this kind, where another child had just died in the family under eclectic treatment, I succeeded in curing. The child coughed up a tube of membrane with the rings of the trachea distinctly impressed on it. This was a case of diphtheritic croup.

Ferrum phos. and *Kali mur.*, so highly recommended by tissue remedy admirers, I have not tried because I have succeeded so well with the above, but

Belladonna has some times served me when in the first or inflammatory or spasmodic stage *Aconite* failed. Here the *Aconite* restlessness and fearful agony was displaced by a condition of as great heat, but there was more of a semi-stupor, twitching and jerking and delirium. Many other remedies might be mentioned, and exceptional cases may call for any one of them according to indications, especially in the diphtheritic form. So far as tracheotomy is concerned, good men can be found to favor or disfavor it. I should not, having had such good results from medication, resort to it early, and would perhaps be charged with failure on account of lateness. But on the other hand, I suspect that many operations claim credit where operation was not at all imperative. In these days of Surgo-phobia the tendency is to a neglect of skillful medical treatment.

Finally: The proper time to treat croup so far as a cure is concerned is when they don't have it. One eminent allopathic authority says, "Appearing, as it does, almost always in children from one to six years old, but sometimes persisting in its occurrence up to puberty, it chiefly depends upon *rickets* or malnutrition, etc." If we had said it depended upon psora, what then? Psora is as easily defined as rickets.

But all hair spliting aside as to names, the principle so often insisted upon of "*treat the patient*," of our school, must be recognized. It would take too much time and space to name the remedies that might be indicated, but must be exhibited in order to not only cure the attack, but cure the tendency thereto.

We will say, however, that that class of remedies having especial influence over psoric, sycotic and syphilitic or phthisical complication should occupy a large place in our attention.

BRONCHITIS.

"Acute Bronchitis is an inflammation of the bronchial tubes, which is usually confined almost entirely to the mucous membrane lining them."

Chronic Bronchitis is the acute form lengthened out, by lack of proper treatment or no treatment at all, and while the cough, expectoration, etc., continue the intense inflammatory symptoms attending the first stage are greatly lessened or absent. If there is a tubercular history of family or not this chronic variety of the disease may go on to tuberculosis.

Either the acute or chronic form may extend downward, implicating the lungs to such a degree that a so-called Broncho-pneumonia may appear.

In these days of what Rosenbach calls "*bacteriophobia*," in which certain "cocci" are insisted on to pronounce a diagnosis, it is hard upon us that we cannot come closer to the mark in this disease, for, as Hare observes, "the micro-organisms infecting the bronchial mucosa are the pneumo coccus, which is the most common; Friedlander's bacillus, the *streptococcus pyogenes*, and the pyogenic staphylococci. The Klebs-Loeffler bacillus is usually present in the bronchitis, which complicates diphtheria. In some cases of bronchitis additional micro-organisms have been found, such as the *Bacillus typhosus*, *Bacillus colo communis* and various forms of fungi. In most instances, however, bronchitis is *polymicrobic* in origin, and it is often impossible to decide what organism is the primary infecting agent."

It is not the provence of this work to give the description and diagnosis of these respiratory affections, and we only allude to the micro-organisms as above to show that for purposes of homœopathic prescribing they amount to little if anything. Even if on microscopical examination tubercle baccilli should be found, the same indications for remedies, according to our art, would have to be applied. Yet for purposes of diagnosis (*naming the disease*), prognosis and hygiene, especially in the latter case (*tuberculosis*) such investigation is very proper and useful. Now in regard to the leading indications for the remedies, we will divide the subject into two general parts, which will practically cover all. And first

ACUTE BRONCHITIS.

In the first or inflammatory stage we will be apt to find our remedies in a list like *Aconite*, *Belladonna* or *Ferrum phos.*

Aconite. Chill followed by synochal fever, high temperature, quick pulse, general dry heat, dry skin, with great restlessness, *fear* and agonized tossing about. There is generally short dry cough, even croupy (in children), and such cases are more often apt to occur after exposure to *dry cold air*. It is best adapted to sanguine, full blooded subjects. If such an attack should occur in a delicate, pale or weakly subject *Ferrum phosphoricum* would generally do better work. With *Ferrum* there is not so much of the nervous excitability as with *Aconite*, but the fever is very great and congestion to the lungs more liable if anything.

Belladonna will follow well either of the two in those cases where *Aconite* has quieted the great excitement, so far as the *anxious* restlessness is concerned, but the heat still continues, though there is a disposition to sweat on the *covered parts*. The disease presents more brain symptoms, such as red eyes, flushed face, *throbbing carotids* and *delirium*, and especially if the child *starts* and jumps in sleep. One of these three remedies will often either check the disease in its first stage or so modify it as to call for one of the following:

Bryonia. Still elevated temperature, great thirst, mouth dry and lips parched, short respiration, dry, hard cough, which hurts the head and chest, splitting headache, and all symptoms greatly aggravated on the least motion, wants to lie perfectly still. It is especially indicated if the trouble extends downward, threatening the lungs and pleura.

Mercurius. The whole mucous membrane catarrhal, but, unlike *Bryonia*, there is great thirst with *moist mouth*, salivation, tongue flabby, showing prints of the teeth upon it, and offensive breath. The fever is still high and there is profuse *sweat, which does not relieve.* The more the sweat the more the suffering.

Chamomilla is especially useful in this stage, especially in children if the heat is accompanied with profuse sweat on the head. The sweat is very hot while that of *Mercurius* may be cold or clammy.

There is great pain and restlessness, child wants to be carried, one cheek *red and hot*, the other pale and cold. The disposition is *ugly*, nothing pleases. Now if these remedies have broken the violence of the attack, but convalescence does not set in satisfactorily, there is danger of it assuming the chronic form.

Sulphur may now come in. There is still some fever which comes and goes in *flashes of heat*, which pass off with a little sweat and debility, there are *faint*, *weak spells*, and generally, or enquiry will often disclose a psoric taint which is *very* apt to stand in the way of satisfactorily indicated drugs. A dose of this remedy may clear up the case and secure prompt recovery or pave the way to the more successful employment of other remedies. If the case seems to settle down into a persistent form of the disease we may have to resort to the following remedies: *Hepar sulphur.*, *Causticum*, *Phosphorus*, *Pulsatilla*, *Kali sulph.*, *Sanguinaria*, *Antimon. tart.*

Hepar sulphur. is indicated when there is a loose, rattling cough, with choking or wheezing breathing. It is not so dry and barking as *Spongia*, still little is expectorated, and the cough is made decidedly worse by exposure to cold air, even if a *hand becomes uncovered.* The cough is also generally < in the early morning hours.

Causticum coughs hard and dry with great SORENESS from larynx down through trachea into the chest. There is apt to be *great hoarseness < in the morning*, and involuntary escape of urine with the cough.

Phosphorus. Larynx so painful he can hardly talk, which aggravates the constant cough. Trembles all over with cough, and it is especially worse in the evening, and *lying on the left side.* Cough hurts and the patient holds the breath and lets it out with a moan because it hurts him so. There is great tendency to extend into the lungs with sense of oppression of the chest. (See Pneumonia.)

Sanguinaria. Coughs hard with circumscribed redness of the cheeks, but its best place is where the disease lingers; a loose cough with offensive expectoration that looks like the patient was running into consumption.

Antimonium tartaricum is almost always loose cough with much *coarse rattling of mucus*, which is so abundant that the patient becomes cyanosed and cannot raise it. This is a serious condition and *Antimonium tart.* will often help. It is particularly found indicated in children and old people. If, notwithstanding the use of this remedy, the rattling and weakness increases, the cyanosis also, until the blood stagnates in the capillaries, the extremities and breath become cold, and the patient gasps fan me, fan harder, *Carbo veg.* is still able to turn the scale in favor of the patient. I have witnessed this result more than once. It is in these cases more of a bronch.-pneumonia than simple bronchitis.

If so far under the preceding remedies the case has improved until the inflammatory symptoms are mainly gone, but there is still considerable cough with loose rattling of mucus which needs clearing up, there are these two remedies that often will do it.

Pulsatilla or *Kali sulphuricum.* The former, if the expectoration is green and bitter, there is bad taste in the mouth, the appetite is poor and the patient is very hungry for cold air, wants cool room or open air. If this does not do all, *Kali sulph.* is its chronic and often follows well on the same indications, of course there are other remedies which may come in according to indication, we cannot tell which one, but the whole materia medica is our armamentarium, and the true homœopath knows how to draw upon it, and use it. When Bronchitis has settled into the chronic form, there may be acute exacerbations that may at times call for the foregoing line of treatment, but a long list of remedies claims our attention; prominent among them are *Sulphur*, *Calcarea carb.* and *Lycopodium*, which Jahr considers a great trio in the order here mentioned, at long intervals apart. *Sanguinaria*, *Kali hydrod.* and *Stannum* form another trio where the expectoration is profuse. *Arsenicum*, *Ipecac* and *Natrum sulph.*, where there are asthmatic complications, will often be very useful. *Kali bich.*, *Hydrastis* and *Coccus cacti*, in profuse stringy expectoration. *Ammonium carb.*, *Cinchona* and *Carbo vegetab.* are often of use in weakened constitutions, especially in aged people. *Hepar sulph.*, *Silicea* and *Tuberculinum* are great in those cases which are profuse and purulent (the expectoration), and especially if every little exposure to cold aggravates the existing conditions. We will mention a few of the many more without attempting to classify them, such as *Alumina*, *Ambra gris.*, *Amm. mur.*, *Iodine*, *Kali carb.*, *Phosphorus*, *Phos. acid.*, *Sepia*, *Lachesis*, *Spongia*, *Drosera*, *Eupat. perf.*, *Balsam peru.*, *Calc. sulph.*, *Grindelia*, *Gummi am.*, *Kreosot.*, *Myosotis*, *Scilla*, *Senega*, *Yerba santa*, etc., and refer for indications first to the articles on *cough* and tuberculosis, then to the repertory and the materia medica, "last and best of all the game."

So far as adjuvants are concerned I have not found medicated inhalations of any advantage, especially when the homœopathic medication was skillfully applied. Avoiding exposure to cold or damp air, and warm, woolen clothing, dry air and sunshine are all that is necessary.

Flax seed emulsion with raisins and lemon juice to flavor is not medicinal, and is soothing to the irritated membranes, and nutritious. It may be used freely and often is very grateful to the patient. It also has a good moral effect and makes the patient feel that he is doing more than when taking only the little pills or watery solution.

ASTHMA.

In giving indications for the remedies for this distressing complaint we have in mind more particularly the variety called *Bronchial Asthma*, or the true asthma which is a pure neurosis, though those varieties which are termed by various authors as "cardiac," "hay," "renal," "thymic," etc., will come, according to symptomatic indications, within the scope of the same therapeutic agents, for, as *Raue* said in regard to organic heart troubles, "the symptoms indicating the curative remedy may often lie outside those which go to make up the pathology of the case." This is a great advantage to the prescriber and does not limit him to understanding the exact pathological condition before he can prescribe. We are often able by such "symptom covering" to cure cases upon which the best pathologists would differ as regards exact conditions. There is perhaps no disease upon which there has been more speculation and less understanding as to its true cause, nature and so forth than this Asthma now under consideration. It is also as difficult to cure. But we have remedies that do often alleviate and sometimes cure, and they are as follows:

Ipecac. Spasmodic form of asthma, *violent contraction*, with rattling or *wheezing* in the bronchial tubes, seems as if would suffocate from constriction, < on motion, and often accompanied with nausea or vomiting.

Arsenicum has just as severe oppression of breathing, is much < at night, especially 1 to 3 A. M. Also on *lying down*, must sit up for fear of suffocation. It is also great < on the *least motion*, particularly on *ascending*, and is > by warmth or warm air, or room. There is often great *anguish*, *restlessness* and thirst for small quantities of water at a time.

These have been the two great remedies from "way back." I used to alternate them, and often with marked relief, but think it is better to give the *Ipecac* first and hold the *Arsenicum* in reserve to follow if necessary, if indicated of course.

Natrum sulphuricum has served me well in a number of cases, when the paroxysms were < or brought on *by damp weather*, which is often the case. Here there is also great rattling and wheezing, and the chest hurts as badly as in the dry cough of *Bryonia*. The patient holds the chest with the hands, it hurts him so to cough. This remedy is oftenest useful in the chronic form, I generally give it in the 30th.

Senega has relieved, and for a long time, some of the worst cases I ever saw. See my "Leaders in Homœopathic Therapeutics" for a fuller description. It must be given low, 5 to 7 drops of the tincture in half glass of water and dessertspoonful dose at intervals corresponding with the violence of the case. I do not know of any work or practice that mentions it for this affection. Now besides these there are many remedies that have done good work. I might mention a few of them, such as

Lobelia which, in addition to the usual difficult

breathing, has a marked *sense of emptiness in the stomach*, and a sensation of a *lump pressing* up into the throat.

Dulcamara may be the remedy when there is much accumulation of mucus, and, like *Natrum sulph.*, is < or brought on by *damp cold weather.*

Aralia racemosa with the general asthmatic symptoms is very prone to come on *after the first sleep.*

Kali carbonica has done beautiful work, especially in elderly people, where the patient had to *sit bent forward* to breathe, and the cough was decidedly < at 3 A. M. Anæmia with bag-like swelling of upper eyelids is strongly corroborative.

Antimon. tartaricum is often beneficial in the cases that become very *loose and rattling*, *coarse rattling*, with inability to expectorate, marked relief follows expectoration.

Lachesis. Attack comes on *after sleep* and *cannot bear anything around throat* or chest. Especially in cardiac cases. To go through all the remedies that *might* become useful in this disease would be to rehearse all that is given in *Raue*, *Lilienthal* and other works on practice. We must refer you to them, and again to the repertories and materia medica.

So far as auxiliaries are concerned there are many of them, such as the different preparations of *Stramonium*, *Nitrate of potash*, *Chloroform*, *Amyl nit.*, etc., but the best of all is a change of location generally to higher altitude and equable climate.

If there is any disease in which a resort to these temporary relief measures would be justifiable it would be in this. I will say in closing that I have succeeded in a few cases in giving complete relief by a long course of treatment along *antipsoric lines*, but not always then. But the greatest hindrance here is that the patients will not consent to a long continued course of treatment; often because they cannot afford it.

So far as those two conditions of diseases, which occur in connection with, or as a consequence of, Bronchitis or Broncho-pneumonia, and called *Bronchiectasis* or *Emphysema*, either interstitial or vesicular, the indications for the remedies are the same, or so nearly so, that it would not be possible to draw very strong lines of distinction. When the case comes to that in any great degree, there is not much hope for a perfect cure, but there is under homœopathic treatment often greater relief and comfort for the patient than under any other.

PERTUSSIS (Whooping Cough).

This affection, now classed among the *infectious diseases*, is to be treated homœopathically just as it was before the *Bacillus pertussis eppendorf* was discovered. In the first stage, when it can hardly be distinguished from a common cold, *Belladonna* is as often indicated as any other remedy. Of course, other remedies may supercede it according to indications. After the whooping stage begins, if there is considerable wheezing and spasmodic coughing with blueness of the face during the paroxysm, also gagging and vomiting, *Ipecac* comes in.

If, instead of becoming loose and wheezing, it continues dry and hard, and hurts the head and stomach or abdomen, is < in the morning or after eating, *Nux vomica* is better. *Belladonna* and *Nux vomica* given early in the case will sometimes so modify it as to need very little medicine afterwards. If the case does not come to us until after the whooping stage is already on, there are a large number of remedies which will have to be chosen from. If the case is in a young child, the cough is violent and the child becomes stiff during the paroxysm, it chokes and swallows as if trying to swallow something down ; it looks pale with pale streaks around mouth and nose rubs its nose, urine profuse or milky after standing awhile, we have a case for *Cina*, which will often do wonders. With *Drosera* the paroxysms are very violent, drawing the whole abdomen spasmodically inward, vomiting of food or mucus, and bleeding from the nose, and sometimes the mouth.

Cuprum metallicum is adapted to one of the worst forms of the disease. The paroxysms are very violent and long continued, *completely prostrating* the patient. The child becomes rigid, turns blue or black in the face, lies as if dead. There is sometimes vomiting after the attack, and rattling of mucus between. It will do best as high as the 200th potency.

Corallium rub. also has a cough so violent that the child *turns purple* or black in the face.

With *Coccus cacti* there is expectoration of large quantities of *viscid*, *stringy* or *albuminous* mucus at the end of each spell of coughing.

Arnica. The child cries before each paroxysm because of the *soreness.* It hurts him so to cough.

Kali bichrom. should be remembered in these cases which, like *Coccus cacti*, has a large amount of stringy mucus expelled. *It hangs down in long strings.*

Veratrum album is one of the chief remedies in the convulsive stage. The child coughs itself into a regular *collapse*, falls over *exhausted* with *cold sweat, especially on the forehead.* It follows well after *Cuprum met.* in these most violent cases.

After this stage is modified or past, the stage of *looseness* or rattling of mucus follows, and may need such remedies as *Pulsatilla* if the expectoration is thick, green and the patient craves fresh, cool air, and is > in a cool room. *Antimon. tart.* if there is much rattling (coarse rattling) of mucus which is difficult to expectorate, especially if the child gets cyanosed from the abundant accumulation When the child coughs it seems as if a cup full of mucus would come but it does not. Sleepiness or coma results. Expectoration relieves. *Carbo veg.* may follow it if the weakness and general blueness from unoxygenized blood, with great hunger for oxygen, *wants to be fanned hard to breathe*, coldness and prostration.

Kali sulph. is useful in those cases in which, after the case is well along, there remains a persistent rattling of mucus, which reminds one of *Pulsatilla*, but it does not finish up the case. *Sulphur* is of course never to be forgotten in any stage, especially in psoric complication, and also in this convalescent stage which we wish to prevent running into a chronic condition leading to permanent lung trouble. For indications see *Cough* and *Tuberculosis*. If the case goes on to a pronounced Bronchitis, Pneumonia or Broncho-pneumonia, the sections on those diseases must be consulted.

The above are the main remedies; there are many others that *may* come in, in fact, do. I will here incorporate with some modifications from "Jahr." "If the paroxysm is preceded by SPASM OF THE GLOTTIS, *Ipec.;* if preceded by ANXIETY, *Cuprum;* if by WEEPING and moaning, *Arn.;* if attended by HEMORRHAGE from the mouth or nose, *Dros.*, *Cina*, *Ipec.;* if VOMITING OF MUCUS without food, *Dros.*, *Verat. alb.*, *Ipec.*, *Tart. em.;* with vomiting of the INGESTA, *Dros.*, *Ipec.*, *Bryon.;* INVOLUNTARY DISCHARGE OF URINE, *Caust.*, *Squill.*, *Verat. alb.;* PAIN IN THE PIT OF STOMACH, *Bry.*, *Nux*, *Dros.;* PAIN IN THE ABDOMEN,

Nux v.; paroxysms of SUFFOCATION, *Ipec.*, *Cupr.*, *Coral.*, *Verat. alb.*, *Arsen.;* PAINS IN THE CHEST, *Bry.*, *Phos.*, *Caust.;* CONVULSIONS OF THE EXTREMITIES, *Cup.;* TETANIC SPASMS, *Cina*, *Cup.*, *Ipec.;* if the attacks end with NOSE-BLEED, *Cina*, *Indigo;* with SNEEZING, *Cina*, *Bell.;* with VOMITING, *Cina*, *Ipec.*, *Cuprum;* with GURGLING down into the abdomen, *Cina;* with long continued SUSPENSION OF BREATHING, *Coral.*, *Cuprum;* with WEEPING or moaning, *Cina*, *Arnica;* with great LASSITUDE or weakness, *Verat. alb.*, *Arsen.;* if BETWEEN the attacks there is rush of blood to the head, *Bell.*, *Bry.;* SORE THROAT with pain, *Carbo veg.*, *Bell.;* VOMITING, also without cough, *Ipec.*, *Puls.*, *Tart. em.*, *Verat. alb.;* a good deal of MUCUS in the air passages, *Cup.*, *Ipec.*, *Cina*, *Tart. em.*, *Seneg.;* SLOW FEVER, with indolence, weakness, weariness, chilliness, thirst, *Verat. alb.*, *Arsenic.;* MILIARIA, especially, *Ipec.*, *Carb. v.*, *Verat. alb.;* BLOATED FACE, especially *over* the eyes, *Kali c.;* finally if the paroxysms of cough set in principally in the EVENING OR AT NIGHT, *Dros.*, *Puls.*, *Carb. veg.;* EARLY IN THE MORNING or AFTER MIDNIGHT, *Kali carb.*, *Hepar*, *Dros.;* EARLY in the morning and FORENOON, *Nux vom.;* AFTER A MEAL, *Nux v.*, *Ipec.*, *Bry.;* WHILE eating, *Clac.*, *Ferr.;* worse in the OPEN AIR, *Carb. v.*, *Rumex*, *Phos.;* worse coming into a WARM ROOM from open air, *Bry.*, *Nat. c.* "For other indications see *repertory* and articles on Cough and Tuberculosis.

The flax seed emulsion is also, as directed under Bronchitis, a good thing, and does not interfere with the most delicate homœopathic remedies.

PNEUMONIA.

However desirable it might be to state exactly whether we had what the text books classify as croupous or lobar, or catarrhal or lobular pneumonia, or whether the micro-organisms, pneumococcus, or streptococcus were present (for in 103 cases of broncho-pneumonia examined by Netter, Weichselbaum and Pierce the streptococcus was found in about 30 and the pneumococcus in 29) for diagnostic purposes, it is not so necessary for therapeutic purposes. And, when we remember that a typical case of lobar pneumonia, as compared with the complicated forms of Broncho-pneumonia, Pleuro-pneumonia, etc., is comparatively rare, we are confirmed in the conclusion that not much success would be likely to follow routine prescribing. Whether the disease (so-called) begins in the lobe and extends upward or outward, or whether it begins in the bronchi and extends downward and outward to the pleura and adjacent organs, is not of so much account as the being able to recognize those symptoms that are peculiar and characteristic in each individual patient, and to choose the homœopathic remedy that most nearly corresponds, in its pathogenesis, with those peculiarities. *Bryonia*, *Phosphorus* or *Sulphur* may be the remedy in either case, and must be chosen largely from indications outside these diagnostic points. Similia Similibus is the guide, no matter in what form or stage of this or any other disease.

The remedies most apt to be indicated in the first, or stage of engorgement, of pneumonia, are *Aconite*, *Belladonna*, *Ferrum phos.* and *Veratrum viride*.

Aconite, if there is a history of chill in cold dry air. The chill is generally pronounced and is promptly followed by high grade inflammatory fever, great heat, dry skin, intense thirst, restlessness, *fear* and anguish, patient tosses about in agony with loud complaints. The expectoration with the cough is tenacious and lumpy, of dark cherry red color. Now if *Aconite* is exhibited in potency from the 6th to the 30th, oft repeated, there will generally follow profuse perspiration and amelioration of all the other symptoms. But if such is not the case after twenty-four hours—

Sulphur 30th once in 2 hours will complement and often conquer the disease in its first stage. These two remedies will abort many cases, if we are called to a case of this character in time, as I can affirm from experience.

Belladonna is to be preferred in this stage, if the fever and heat is fully as great as that of the *Aconite* case, but the patient is more stupid, not so anguished, but jerks and twitches in sleep, is delirious, the eyes are very red, the face dark red and bloated, especially upper lip; the carotids throb and beat visibly, and instead of the universally hot, dry skin there is sweat on the *covered* parts; the blood seems to mount to the brain as well as the chest, and it is sometimes, especially in children, difficult to tell whether the brain or lung is the center of the trouble, from outward signs. The *Belladonna* case is more apt to run into that condition which is called typhoid pneumonia.

Ferrum phos. seems to me to stand midway between *Aconite* and *Belladonna*, for while it does not present the excitement and fear of *Aconite*, on the other hand it does not produce so strong brain symptoms as *Belladonna*. I have found it of most service in pale anæmic subjects, who are subject to flushes of heat and redness of the face, and to local congestions generally. It certainly does fine work in such subjects in this stage of the disease. In regard to

Verat. viride I wrote in "Leaders" that at one time it had a great reputation in the first or congestive stage of inflammatory diseases, and especially in those organs coming under control of the pneumogastric nerve, viz., pharynx, œsophagus, stomach and heart. For a time the journals fairly bristled with reported cures of pneumonia, and its curative power was attributed to the influence of the remedy to control the action of heart and pulse. It was claimed that if we could control the quickened circulation so as to decrease the amount of blood forced into the congested lung, that you thereby gave the lung a chance to free itself of the existing engorgement.

It looked plausible, and certainly in many cases remarkable cures were effected, and that in a short time. I was a young physician and thought I had found a prize in this remedy. But one day I left a patient, apparently relieved by it of an acute attack of pneumonia, to go to a town five miles distant, and when I returned found my patient dead. Then I watched others so treated, and found every little while a patient with pneumonia dropping out *suddenly* when they were reported better. Now we don't hear so much of *Veratrum viride* as the greatest remedy for the first stage of this disease. What was the matter? 1st. It was (like other fads) used too indiscriminately. 2d. It is not desirable (it is wrong) to control or *depress the pulse* regardless of all the other conditions. 3d. The patients who had weak hearts were killed by this powerful heart depressant. A quickened circulation is salutary in all inflammatory diseases, and is evidence that the natural *power* to resist disease, is there and at work. The pulse will come to its normality when the cause of its disturbance is removed and should never be forced to do so until then. Here is a common fault of the old school, notwithstanding their cry of "*Tolle causam.*" So I find fault with Guernsey's key-note, "Great activity of the arterial system; very quick pulse." Next to *Digitalis*, *Veratrum viride slows* the pulse, as is abundantly shown in the provings. If quick pulse is ever the result of this remedy, it is a secondary or re-actionary effect, like the sleeplessness of *Opium* or the constipation of cathartics. So it seems to me that as an antiphlogistic (forgive me) it must go into the shade with the once vaunted *Digitalis*.

Gatchell writes (pocket-book): "This is the most important remedy in the stage of engorgement, to which its use must be limited. In my own experience and in that of others, it has apparently cut short oncoming attacks of pneumonia. It must be given early, immediately following the chill. It is of no avail after hepatization has begun. Again, if it produces nausea reduce the dose. Watch the action to *avoid cardiac depression*." I should object to the wholesale assertion that this is *the* most important remedy, for the most important remedy is the homœopathically indicated one, and it is not *Verat. viride* always by any means. I fully concur with him in the necessity of watching its action and for the same reason. I do know of one good characteristic indication for its use, not only in congestion of the lungs, but in other congestions also, viz., *the well defined red streak running right through the middle of the tongue.*

It has been repeatedly verified. So while it is true that it may be able to cut short oncoming cases of this disease, I should be sure one of the other more safe remedies was not indicated before I would use it, especially in weak heart cases.

In the second stage, that of hepatization, we have quite a long list of remedies. Prominent among them are *Bryonia*, *Phosphorus*, *Iodine*, *Rhus tox.*, *Hyoscyamus*, *Lachesis*, *Sanguinaria*, *Mercury*, *Chelidon.*, *Ant. tart.*, *Lycopod.*, *Opium*, *Kali carb.*, *Carbo veg.*, *Arsenicum*, *Sulphur*, *Calcarea carb.* and others. We say others because this list must be added to in peculiar cases, and the whole materia medica must be the resort of the homœopathic physician in all cases, and the name of the disease has little to do with the selection.

Bryonia is very often indicated after the remedies

for the stage of engorgement have done all they can. It is especially in cases of pleuro-pneumonia that it is most useful. The fever still continues being only partially controlled by the former treatment, the breathing is short, expiration shorter than inspiration, the patient wants to lie perfectly still on the *painful side*, as the least motion aggravates all the symptoms; there is great thirst for large draughts of water, with corresponding dryness of mouth, and lips, which are dry and cracked, or parched (only exceptionally there is no thirst), the expectoration is generally tenacious and sometimes falls in round jelly-like lumps of a yellow or soft brick shade. It is the stage of the exudation, or the second stage of the inflammatory process, and if given in nick of time, in not too low a potency, say, 12th to 200th, will often finish the case, promoting absorption and all If it does not complete the case, but has well started it toward cure, no remedy follows it so well (generally) as *Sulphur*, which will often do the rest and prevent chronic conditions following. The pains of *Bryonia* are characteristically *stitching* pains, which, occurring as they do in serous membranes, show that the pleura is involved.

Phosphorus is very different. There is greater oppression of the chest, feels as if there were a load pressing it down. The parenchyma of the lung is the centre of action and the pleura not so much involved, if at all; the expectoration is often profuse, and when falling on paper, on a hard surface, will break and fly like batter; the temperature is very high with circumscribed red cheeks (*Sang.*), cough hurts and makes him tremble and is worse lying on the left side; the patient moans or grunts with every breath, and suppresses the cough by it, just as long as he can because it hurts him so. *Phosphorus* attacks by preference the lower right lung or lobe. It may be indicated by the symptoms at the beginning of the stage of hepatization, when it puts a stop to the further progress of the disease, but its more brilliant effect is when the stage of hepatization is completed and we want to break it up and promote resolution. Here it has no equal. Under its action the hitherto restless patient, will, (in the 30th, 200th or 1000th potency), sink into a sweet sleep, profuse perspiration will set in, and with the waking we are in full tide of convalescence, the expectoration becomes free and easy, the mind tranquil, and, in short, all the violence of the storm is past. A dose of *Sulphur* or *Lycopodium* may be needed to finish the case, and will be given according to indications, of course. We will next mention

Iodine. Kafka says "at the beginning when the disease localizes itself." Well, if that was all, what a "dead easy" time we would have of it. Gatchell does better than that when he says—"It replaces *Bryonia* in a certain class of subjects. There is fever with high temperature, but an abscence of the pleuritic pains of *Bryonia.*" The *class of subjects* is a large factor in the *Iodine* case. It is the subject that is spare, dark complexioned (brunette), dark eyes, subject to scrofulous affections of the glands, especially goitre. The fever does not give way to *Aconite*, but continues with great general nervous and irritated manifestations, even when the case has gone on to a chronic form. Absorption does not take place, and the patient emaciates greatly, though he may want to eat and feels better while doing so. In such cases *Iodine* may do more than any other remedy. My observation is that it does better low, say, the 2d trit., than higher. *Lycopod.* follows well and is adapted to the same kind of temperament.

Rhus toxicod. If the case assumes a typhoid tendency, as shown by the tongue with its dryness and triangular red tip, and the excessive restlessness which keeps the patient tossing about, and the sensorium is blunted with low delirium. If this remedy does not, within a reasonable time, modify the symptoms and the delirium increases, also the stupor until the case is unconscious, no remedy surpasses *Hyoscyamus*. I am quite sure this remedy (*Hyos.*) is not so well and favorably known as it should be in this disease.

Lachesis, if the *Rhus* and *Hyos.* fail, will do good work if the stupor increases, the weakness also; the patient is unable to put out the tongue, it trembles and catches behind the lower teeth when trying to protrude it, showing great weakness, there is great oppression of breathing with aversion to having anything touching the chest or throat, pulse weak and intermittent, with general aggravation of the whole case after sleep. Left-sided pneumonia oftenest calls for this remedy.

Opium is sometimes of great use in old topers, where there is sopor with heavy breathing, even stertorous; the whole body bathed in a hot sweat, and the patient complains of the bed feeling too hot.

Sanguinaria. Typhoid pneumonia, second and third stage, extreme dyspnœa, tough, rust colored sputa, face and hands cold, or the opposite hot and burning (*Sulph.*), circumscribed redness and burning heat of the cheeks, especially in the afternoon.

Arsenicum and *Carbo veg.* are both indicated in those desperate cases that resist the above remedies.

Arsenicum is most likely to come in after *Rhus tox.* If the restlessness continues and added to it the weakness and prostration increases. There is great thirst for small quantities at a time, burning pain and heat in chest (*Sang.*), feels better from warmth and is worse from 1 to 3 A. M. generally.

Carbo veg. Cough by spells or no cough; if cough with rattling but too weak to expectorate (*Ant. tart.*); *Ant. tart.* has failed; hippocratic face, nose pinched and cold; lips, hands, feet and skin blue and cold, breath cold, dyspnœa great, wants to be fanned, can't get oxygen enough, vital force almost expended. I have seen several such cases come out under *Carbo veg.*, re-action setting in so that other remedies that did not act satisfactorily will now take hold and do better work *Antimon. tart.* is often of great utility where the case has gone into what might be called the "loosening up" stage. The chest seems full of mucus with coarse rattling and cough which seems as though it must bring up large quantities, but it does not; the patient becomes cyanotic from want of oxygen, which the great accumulation of mucus shuts out, there seems to be lack of strength to expectorate, even threatened paralysis of the lungs; fits of suffocation. This is the condition that precedes the desperate stage of *Carbo veg.* and may save the patient from it. It is oftenest found in children and very old people.

Ipecac., which also has great accumulation of mucus, is again useful in children, but the oppression of breathing is accompanied with squeaky *wheezing* breathing instead of the coarse rattling of *Ant. tart.*

Mercurius, *Chelidonium* and *Kali carb.* are a trio that go well in company. These remedies all suit cases of pneumonia with bilious complication.

Mercurius, if there are with the oppressed breathing stitches in right chest through from scapulæ; cough, first dry, afterward attended with bloody expectoration, great tenderness in region of stomach, and, especially, liver; mouth and tongue moist, but tongue large, flabby, showing imprint of the teeth, great thirst and *profuse sweat without relief*, worse at night and when lying on right side.

Kali carbon. also has stitching pains running through lower part of right side, and the cough is worse toward 3 A. M., there is wheezing and rattling breathing, pulse often intermitting. It is often a complementary to *Bryonia* when that remedy has only partially relieved the stitching pains. Of course *Mercurius* and *Kali carb.* cases are oftener the ones in which bilious or pleuritic complications are markedly present.

Chelidonium has pain under the right shoulder-blade and in the liver, with marked jaundice, yellow face and skin, tongue coated yellow at the base (*Merc. prot.*), yellow urine and very yellow stool, yellow as gold, or very white stools.

All these remedies have done good work in such cases, and have done it both in low and high potencies. For the use of *Kali iodatum* see my "Leaders in Homœopathic Therapeutics," page 118, third edition. I will not repeat that here as I have not had occasion to use the remedy in pneumonia, though others have and with beautiful results.

Now when we come to the third stage, the stage of *gray hepatization*, which follows that of red hepatization, when "the acute inflammation in the lung has passed by, and nature begins the task of clearing away the products of the disease, which is accomplished by the cells, which have been extravasated, undergoing fatty degeneration and granular change, while the fibrin undergoes softening. During this stage of resolution the exudation is gotten rid of by absorption and expectoration. Finally the air cells are freed from the exudate which has been filling them, the epithelium lining them is reproduced, and recovery results." (Hare). To hasten this most desirable result, or to secure it when nature in her unaided efforts is unable to accomplish it, we have another class of remedies, among which may be mentioned *Sulphur*, *Calcarea*, *Lycopod.*, *Hepar*, *Sanguinaria*, *Psorinum*, *Tuberculinum* and others.

Sulphur has always, and perhaps always will,

occupy first place here, as indeed it does in many other diseases where the process of absorbing the effusions which are the result of acute or even chronic inflammation is desired. It is especially useful if after the violence of the storm of active inflammation is passed there remain fitful flashes of fever ending in debilitating sweats, faintness or weakness. These are the cases which do not finish up their stages well, and it is generally on account of *psoric* taint in the patient. Hence relapses occur again and again on account of deficient vital re-action. We have not only the *disease* to deal with, but a condition of the *patient* which existed beforehand, perhaps all his life. Such patients will have *Sulphur* symptoms in general. The case will not clear up, the apparently indicated remedy does not act satisfactorily. It may be a *Sulphur* subject, viz.—lean, stoop-shouldered persons, who walk or sit stooped, standing especially aggravates. Skin eruptions are present, or were in his usual condition, but especially if they have disappeared during the progress of the disease. If this latter is the case probably a restoration of the skin eruption will be necessary before there will be satisfactory improvement or cure.

Burning in chest, skin or locally in many places, and especially of the feet, which must be stuck out of bed to cool them. Weakness, or weak, empty or gone feeling at the stomach, especially worse at 11 A. M.; white tongue with very red tip and borders, bright redness of the lips as if the blood would burst through, or redness of any and all orifices. All or any of these symptoms present will point to this great antipsoric, and when we remember its strong powers of absorption, we may then readily understand why *Sulphur* leads the van in the list as a "finisher" of the case.

Calcarea carb. stands for a different class of subjects, viz., the *leucophlegmatic.* "Fair, fat and *flabby.*" There is characteristically *coldness* instead of burnings. I cannot do better here for want of space than again to refer you to my "Leaders in Hom. Therap.," 3d Ed., page 60, to get the picture. The case continues to cough and expectorate, $<$ in the morning; the external chest becomes sensitive to touch and sore. Sensation in feet and legs as if she had on cold, damp stockings; night sweats, general, and especially local sweats, to which the patient may have been subject all her life. She was sweaty headed as a child. Now *Calcarea* may save this case from running on to consumption if it is given properly.

Lycopodium is one of the best remedies for the later stages of typhoid or neglected pneumonia, and is especially indicated when there is copious expectoration, the parenchyma of the lung sounds full of mucus, there is often circumscribed redness of the cheeks, especially at 4 to 8 P. M.; often red sand in the urine and fan-like motion of the alæ nasi. It is often the best remedy to finish the cure where there have been liver complications such as we noticed under *Mercurius*, *Chelidon.* and *Kali carb.* Of course, if we have the flatulent condition so characteristic of this remedy it is additional indication for its use.

In the use of these remedies (*Sulph.*, *Calc.* and *Lyc.*) I never use at this stage anything below the 30th potency, and often use much higher. *Sulph.* 55m., Fincke, and *Lycopod.* 6m., Jenichen, are favorites with me.

Sanguinaria is often of greatest utility when the profuse expectoration becomes *very offensive* to the patient. It also has circumscribed redness of the cheeks, and acts especially well on the right upper lung. I have used the 200th with good results, but have also seen the most prompt and radical results from the 2d trituration of the alkaloid.

Psorinum has profuse green expectoration and the patient is very *despondent*, thinks he is never going to get well, and sweats from weakness on the least exertion or when asleep.

Tuberculinum is useful in patients of tubercular history, when the patient complains of feeling as if he had taken a new cold on the least exposure, and it has erratic pains like *Pulsatilla*, appearing now here, now there, in different parts of the body.

Pulsatilla will sometimes close up the case when the expectoration becomes thick, profuse, green and bitter or offensive tasting, and the patient feels chilly, yet cannot bear the atmosphere of a close warm room.

Kali sulph. where the expectoration is like that of *Pulsatilla*, and the aggravations and ameliorations are similar. It seems to be what we call the "chronic" of *Pulsatilla*.

Hepar sulphur. often helps where there remains a wheezy condition, and the least cold air makes the cough worse. This combination of *Lime* and *Sulphur* is wonderful, and while it has symptoms similar to each, has new ones of its own. It is a remedy well worth bearing in mind in these cases.

Now in regard to auxiliary measures.

In regard to stimulants so much vaunted now-a-days by many, the best stimulant is the homœopathic remedy. Hare (old school) says; "It is, however, a fatal mistake to think that every patient suffering from this disease should be stimulated." He recommends in some cases Aromatic spirits of *Ammonia*, and Hoffman's Anodyne. And here is something for those quasi homœopaths who are so anxious and fearful that the homœopathic remedy will not do all that is possible. The same old school authority says—"At the present time it has become fashionable for physicians (of the old school, of course) to administer *Strychnine* as a cardiac stimulant throughout the whole course of pneumonia. This is an *abuse* of a good remedy, *Strychnine* is not a direct cardiac stimulant. It increases the activity of the heart by rallying the nervous system and acting as an indirect whip to the circulation. If it is persisted in it soon loses its so-called stimulant effects, and is apt to produce a condition of nervous irritation, particularly in the aged, which may be quite distressing. Its constant use deprives the physician of a valuable remedy for meeting critical moments in the course of the disease." Some of us would do well to take heed to such words from high allopathic authority. If we do not *know our homœopathic similimum* and our case seems on the verge of cardiac collapse it might be excusable to use it, not otherwise. I have seen a desperate case where there was obstructed flow of the blood through the lung from organic, or valvular disease of long standing, markedly helped by *Digitalis*, low, and it is in just such cases that homœopathic indications will be found for it. The relief was wonderful and the pneumonia cured, while, of course, the valvular condition still remained. So far as local applications are concerned, I prefer to use warm dry ones instead of poultices I do not believe that inunction of turpentine and lard is of any use. So far as oxygen inhalations are concerned, I again agree with Hare (allopathic) that their value is problematical. If I used it I would not dam up the patient's nostrils with a nozzle, but let him breathe it mixed with common air as it escaped through the rubber tube or glass nozzle about the nose or lips of the patient. In regard to forcing the temperature of the patient down by antipyretic drugs it is not necessary, it is damaging. Let me quote again from old school authority (Hare), and I do so freely for the reason that I find many so-called homœo's frightened to death by a high temperature. Quotation, "There is overwhelming clinical and experimental evidence to show that the use of these drugs materially diminishes the vital resistance of the patient, decreases the ability of his blood to convey oxygen to his tissues, reduces its ability to destroy infecting micro-organism, lowers vascular tone, depresses the heart, and is altogether evil in its influence, probably also diminishing the elimination of toxic materials by the kidneys, and certainly giving these organs the additional labor of eliminating the antipyretic, which, perchance, may be irritating to them."

I quote thus at length from this old school authority because that even in that school, in the abscence of such therapeutic measures as abound in Homœopathy, they have no confidence in the process of treatment that seeks to control the disease process by simply striking at the temperature. Under homœopathic treatment the temperature will take care of itself as the patient comes under the influence of the indicated remedy. And it is so with every other so-called disease. Now in regard to cough remaining after pneumonia, again the remedy that covers the case "in toto" will take care of the cough, too. I have known physicians to resort to Dover's powder, cocaine, paregoric, or the newer drug, heroin, for this cough, claiming that it was better for the patient, though unhomœopathic, than to wear himself out with coughing. If the doctor is not able to select the right remedy (homœopathic) for this as well as other conditions, let him do it, but let him never claim that Homœopathy is inadequate, for the inadequacy is in him and not in Homœopathy. Pneumonia is often the beginning of the road to phthisis pulmonalis in subjects predisposed to it, and we might give the remedies that are most appropriate for it, but will do so when coming to treat of that fell destroyer.

PLEURITIS.

In this disease, if it is ushered in by one, or repeated chills, and especially if it occurs after exposure to dry cold air, followed by high fever, great thirst, quick pulse, dry, hot skin, anxious restlessness, agonized tossing about, sticking pains in chest, dry hacking cough, *Aconite* is the remedy. If this remedy is given in the 12th or 30th once an hour to three hours, according to violence of the symptoms, it will often check the disease in from 24 to 48 hours. But if we are called in too late and the stage of effusion is begun or the *Aconite* does not remove all the trouble the next remedy is generally *Bryonia* when the sharp stitching pain continues, and the thirst and fever also; the pain and suffering is aggravated on the *least motion*, and the patient feels better lying on the painful side; the tongue is coated white. No remedy acts more positively on the serous membranes, and it may finish the case, even to promote the effusion, which *Aconite* could not do.

If the case seems to be progressing favorably this remedy may be used right along for days, or as long as improvement continues.

Mercurius may follow well after, or even be preferred, if in syphilitic or rheumatic subjects we have the pain persisting after the fever is somewhat reduced, the pain continues notwithstanding *copious sweats which do not relieve;* thirst with moist tongue, which is enlarged, flabby and shows imprint of teeth, gums also swollen and an offensive smell from the mouth. It is especially useful when with the cough there are stitching pains through to the back in region of lower right lung. But if you do not have the Mercurial mouth and the point is in the same locality running through to the back, or it may be in the left side, and the cough is worse at 3 A. M., *Kali carbonica* will outrank *Mercury* and is complementary to *Bryonia*.

Rhus toxicod. should be considered when the tongue grows dry with a triangular red tip and the sensorium becomes more dull like typhoid form of fever, the patient being very restless, wanting to change position often, and especially if the case has a history of exposure to wet or from straining, wrestling, lifting, etc. There may be fever blisters on lips and around mouth. Now if neither one of the foregoing remedies avail we may suspect some psoric complications in the case and may exhibit

Sulphur, especially if the case seems to get a little better and relapses again and again. The fever comes and goes in fitful flashes, followed by spells of sweat and debility. Again the patient complains of burning, especially of the feet, which must be uncovered or stuck out of bed. There may be diarrhœa < in the A. M. The lips are not so dry, cracked or blistered as in *Bryonia* and *Rhus tox.*, but are very red, sometimes vermillion red. This remedy will, when these symptoms are present often finish up the case, even to absorption of large quantities of effusion. It should be watched "out" for in connection with any of the other remedies and may be interpolated with advantage in any and all stages of the disease.

Very few cases will fail to respond to the above remedies unless serious complications exist.

If in exceptional cases there are strong head symptoms as delirium, high fever and red hot skin, thirst, throbbing carotids and sweat on covered parts while uncovered parts remain hot and dry, the patient moaning and twitching in sleep, all worse at 3 P. M. or A. M., and *Aconite* does not modify these high grade inflammatory symptoms, *Belladonna* will often do it or so modify them that *Bryonia*, *Mercurius*, *Rhus* or *Sulphur* will again come in to take the case along when the stage of effusion is established in spite of the above treatment, or we are not called in in time to prevent it, and the process of absorption is delayed if the patient shows signs of increasing prostration to an alarming degree. If the thirst is for cold water in small and often repeated quantities, there is great dyspnœa, and little pain which motion greatly aggravates, increasing the prostration and the dyspnœa, notwithstanding the patient suffers great anguish and restlessness, so that he wants to be moved or carried from room to room, or place to place, and especially if all is aggravated at night, 1 to 4 A. M., *Arsenicum album* must be given and will often change the whole aspect for the better in a few hours. Such cases will be often found in cachectic persons, drunkards, malarial subjects and in pyothorax.

Carbo veg. complements it if there is great prostration, sunken hippocratic face, general coldness and blueness, and there is rattling respiration and dyspnœa with desire to be fanned hard to help the breathing. These two last remedies of course come into those desperate cases which have defied the former remedies.

When the disease action spreads and involves the lungs and bronchi, as it sometimes does, constituting a case of pleuro-pneumonia, which it sometimes does, though it is oftener the other way in my experience, *i. e.*, beginning in the lung first; the pneumonic remedies must come into the case, viz., *Phosphorus*, bronchitis with severe cough, which is worse in the evening, and when lying on the left side, dyspnœa with a sense of heaviness in the chest. It generally comes in the later stages of the disease with purulent infiltration, and in flat chested people of a consumptive build. It must be used in those cases which "hang fire" in the process of convalescence, after improvement sets in and consumption threatens, or in those cases which show decided tubercular signs, and just here is where *Tuberculinum* may do good work in cases having a decided tubercular family history. I have seen such cases do well on a dose of this remedy once a week, interpolated with the other indicated remedies, just as we give *Psorinum* in psoric cases, and now we mention *Psorinum* in this connection, it must also be used if the symptoms are present and may be preferred before *Tuberculinum.*

Tartar. emetic., regarded by Kafka as specific at the commencement of pleuro-pneumonia, has great dyspnœa, must sit up to breathe, sometimes nausea and vomiting, but is more especially called for when there is much coarse rattling of mucus in the tubes, they are so loaded as to threaten suffocation and it cannot be expectorated, cyanosis appears and death will quickly come if not relieved. Here this remedy is wonderfully efficacious if relief is possible. If it fails the choice is next generally *Carbo veg.*, according to indications above given under that remedy. The *Veratrum* is useful in collapse with prostration, general coldness and cold sweat, especially on the *forehead.* It may not cure the case, but will often bring on a reaction, as will also *Arsenicum* and *Carbo veg.*, much better than the hypodermics of Strychnia of the old school. I have seen desperate cases recover under these remedies, skillfully applied. More than once nurses who had been used to the Strychnia expressed their astonishment at the result, which so seldom had been accomplished under that treatment.

If pleuritis occurs after mechanical injuries the first stage will often have to be controlled with *Aconite*, *Bryonia* or the other remedies above mentioned, but sooner or later *Arnica* must come in, and, being in itself a powerful absorbent, will finish it up, or, if not, is well followed by *Sulph. acid*, which is also a fine remedy to cure *ecchymoses*, the result of trauma. The indications aside from the history of injury for *Arnica* are aching or bruised sensation, torpidity even to sepsis, dry, cold extremities, head hot, remaining body cool, and soreness general as if the bed lain upon were too hard.

If in addition to the pleuritic inflammation there is pain in the intercostal muscles, the result or not of strain, *Rhus tox.*, *Ranunculus bulb.* or *Cimicifuga*, according to indicating symptoms, are often very efficient.

Cantharis must be given if the characteristic urinary symptoms are present, for it also has profuse serous exudation, frequent cough, dyspnœa, and profuse sweats.

I will only give a passing mention to *Calcarea carb.* or *phos.*, which has caused a rapid subsidence of pleuritic exudation, and *Lycopod.*, which is exceedingly valuable in the lithic acid diathesis suffering from pleuritis or in any other disease.

Pyæmic cases will often get great help from our *Hepar sul.*, *Calc. sul.*, *Silicea*, etc., and, indeed, individual cases may call for remedies not mentioned here. *Symptom correspondence* must not be ignored, and no amount of pathological speculation or routine prescribing can improve such prescribing. While the fact remains that we only exceptionally have a case of pneumonia, pleuritis or bronchitis pure and simple, but on the other hand do have a complication of two or three together, it is obvious that the names of disease have little to do after all with prescribing, I mean good prescribing; but the case in its entirety, the *patient*, with all his individuality and idiosyncrasies, must be taken into account. So far as auxiliary measures are concerned, I prefer warm to cold applications to the chest unless the patient prefers cold, being more relieved by them. Surgical interference is in some cases imperative, and here is the best chance for the surgeon to get good results where homœopathic treatment has prepared the patient for operation. Surgeons as a rule are not good prescribers, I believe, for it is hardly possible that one head can contain a thorough knowledge at once of advanced surgery and our vast materia medica and therapeutics. But the two (physician and surgeon) working like true yoke-fellows together will be able to accomplish more than either can separately.

PULMONARY TUBERCULOSIS.

Whether called this name (as by Hare), pulmonary phthisis (by Butler), or old fashioned phthisis pulmonalis makes little difference. The same microbe is there, according to the science of bacteriology, getting in his work. This disease is now classed as infectious, because it is believed to take place as a primary process through the entrance of the bacillus by the respiratory passages, or, secondarily, as the result of the transference of the bacillus from some primary focus by the blood-vessels or lymphatics. But we, with Rosenbach, of Berlin (when applied to the theme of infectious disease), enter the objection that it is *wrong* to ascribe the origin of all these affections exclusively to the action of microbes. It must be demonstrated that the mere presence of minute organisms in disease is not sufficient to explain the nature and the mechanism of the affection. It must be emphasized that much study must be applied to the investigation of circumstances, which, in the presence of the so-called generator of the disease, only furnish the essential preliminary conditions for its successful action. So far it has been quite falsely presumed that the conditions favoring the thriving of micro-organisms should be looked for solely in their external (exoteric) circumstances. It was assumed, for instance, that the cholera bacillus might be transmitted, but would not be capable of infecting because it would not find the preliminary conditions necessary to its development in the soil. It was assumed that the height of the ground-water (*Grundwasser*) is in a similar relation to the developement of the typhoid bacillus, and that certain conditions of the ground-water favor an increase of the typhoid germs, and with it the outbreak of an epidemic. These facts are surely correct, and it is quite conceivable from the standpoint of the struggle of the organisms that conditions which have become more favorable for the existence of a species enhance its faculty of becoming harmful. This, however, does not yet account for the second factor, the weakening of the attacked organism—very wrongly, in our opinion, since generally not the intensity of the pathogenic organism plays the principal part in the infection of the individual, but the *predisposition*, *i. e.*, the weakened condition of the attacked, or a coincidence of both factors. "Activity of bacteria is certainly and inseparably combined with the origin of certain diseases, but it is only a cause of disease when the indispensable preliminary condition (a weak or weakened organism), is present."

It would be more nearly correct, therefore, and would avoid misunderstanding not to use the term "*cause*" for the role played by the microbes in the origin of disease, and to say, instead, the cause of the disease is the *weak body*, whereas, the impulse to affection, *i. e.*, the production of an altered condition of internal functions, is given by the presence of certain micro-organisms." (One would almost think he heard Hahnemann talking). Again Rosenbach, "Experiment and the predominating study of test-tube cultures have served to *obscure* the true state of affairs, since they tend most unjustifiably to minimize the individual predisposition of the infected person, and to overestimate the ability of the microbes to infect in every instance. It is true in producing experimental infectious disease in which the microorganisms from cultures are introduced in great numbers and directly into the circulation the effect of the microbes alone is in evidence, but it is manifest against an almost defenseless enemy." So it would seem from this above reasoning that Hering, Hahnemann & Co., were quite right in turning their therapeutic guns in such a direction as would expel the enemy outside the citadel by *treating the patient* instead of the disease. But we think the same treatment is operative by restoring the partially overcome vital force to its normality and expel so-called disease, even after it has succeeded in gaining a lodgment. And now to quote once more from the above authority as to the treatment. "The possibility of certain substance (remedies) shielding, or at least assisting, the attacked animal organism is by no means excluded. On the contrary, that they can do so, and why, are clearly shown above. *They must be capable of being absorbed by the living cell, thereby increasing its power of resistance* (potency). They must remain in the body so long as the inimical agency is still active, and must, therefore, be supplied, not irregularly, at any period, but as nearly as possible at periods corresponding to the activity of the foreign agent (repetition of dose). Such remedies must be of *weak concentration*, *so as not to paralize the activity of the living cell*, while at the same time they aid in shielding it against renewed attacks of foreign cells by making *untenable* the vital conditions necessary for the activity of these assailants." It doesn't seem after such talk that Rosenbach could stand very strongly against the homœopathic preparations in regard to dose or repetition of it. All this quotation is in order to show how even an old school physician high in authority takes position against the "overgrowth of bacteriology," and that the eagerness of bacteriologists to transfer decisions from the bedside to the laboratory is not scientific, that it is impossible to regulate etiology, diagnosis and therapy, endemics and epidemics, individual and general prophylaxis, according to such an artificial scheme, but that full allowance for the requirements of actual conditions can only be judged by those who are present at the bedside, etc.

All this is interesting to read from old school authority and, we, who are in the habit of prescribing remedies according to our law, have had occasion enough to observe that the bacteria so active under favorable surroundings become less so, or inactive and harmless, under the changes wrought by the homœopathic remedy.

"It is not long since it was almost universally thought that subacute pulmonary tuberculosis was an utterly hopeless and incurable disease. At present we know that it is in many instances a readily curable affection. Further we know that hundreds of persons have the disease and get well without knowing that they have ever had it. It is manifest, however, that only those cases can recover in which the disease is not far advanced, and in which the *vital resistance of the individual* can be maintained at such a level that the protective processes of combat and repair, already described, can be carried out to completion" (Hare).

This we believe to be very true, and that the proper and timely exhibition of the indicated drug, according to well known homœopathic principles, is *the* important and indispensable agent with which to establish and maintain this "*vital resistance of the individual*," and it makes no difference at what stage of the disease it must be the remedy *indicated by the symptoms* at the time, that must be used. Cough, dyspnœa, fever, sweat, chill, loss of weight, anæmia, sputum, etc., each and all go to make the picture which must find its similar counterpart in the corresponding remedy, whether in the incipient or advanced stage where caseation, ulceration, and hæmoptysis are about to close the scene. It is impossible to say what remedy will be called for in any individual case at the beginning, but we will very often find one of the following list indicated:

Sulphur, *Psorinum*, *Tuberculinum*, *Hepar sulphur.*, *Calcarea ost.*, *Phosphorus*, *Arsenicum alb.*, *Sanguinaria.*

Sulphur is perhaps oftener indicated here in the

first stage than any other remedy. Generally the exciting cause is some acute affection like laryngitis, bronchitis, pneumonia, pleurisy, etc., and on account of tuberculous tendency of the patient convalescence "hangs fire." The hepatization, pleuritic effusion, or other effects of the acute trouble do not "clear up." Now, as is well known, *Sulphur* is a powerful absorbent, or, as Father Hering used to say, "a finisher." If given early (on indications, of course), the chronic troubles consequent on only imperfectly cured cases will be avoided. Symptoms indicating are—the *pulse* and *temperature* do not go and *stay* down, there are hot flushes of fever by spells, and this is followed by debilitating sweats; strength and appetite comes slowly or none at all, while the patient still is thirsty, as the characteristics put it—"*drinks much, eats little.*" The circulation is weak and uneven, as is manifest in the alternately cold and *hot burning feet*, which must be *put out of bed to cool them.* If the patient is psoric, which is generally the case, the eczema or other skin troubles have disappeared during the sickness and do not re-appear. Psoric history is always a pointer toward *Sulphur.* "*Nightly suffocating attacks, wants doors and windows open.*" Cough may be dry or loose and rattling. Great sense of weakness in the chest when talking or reading (*Stann.*). Pain running through left upper chest to scapula (*Myrtus*, *Pix liquida*, *Theridion* and *Tuberc.*). *Morning diarrhœa driving out of bed*, if present, is a strong indication for *Sulphur.* These symptoms are often present in such cases, and the remedy should not be given too low or too often repeated to get the best results. Or if you *must* repeat, do so for a day or two and then give *Sac. lac.* and wait for results.

Psorinum should never be forgotten in an *unquestionably psoric subject* If *Sulphur* fails where there is in the history of the case a supressed eruption, scabies, herpes, eczema, etc., *Psorinum* is the next remedy to be thought of; and especially if the poor health of the patient dates back to some former acute affection. The patient has never been well since that time (*Carbo veg.*). The *Psorinum* patient is very sensitive to *cold air or change of weather*. Wears a fur cap, overcoat or shawl even in the hottest weather (*Hep.*), is easily affected by stormy weather, and is restless for days before a storm or during a thunder storm.

There is great weakness, debility, even though there is no organic disease perceptible. Sweats on slight exertion or at night, and is discouraged or hypochondriacal to a degree not surpassed by any other remedy. *The excretions generally are offensive;* sometimes of a carrion-like odor. The hair is lustreless, mats at the tips and tangles easily, and the skin or eruptions *itch intolerably*, < at night or in *warmth of the bed.* There is short or oppressed breathing, *relieved lying down*, riding and moderate exercise. Cough, dry, hacking, and for a long time until expectoration occurs, then there is THICK, GREEN PUS-LIKE expectoration. *Cough returns every winter* (*Cham.*). Dr. Halleck, of Saranac Lake, lauds this remedy very highly after much experience and observation.

It does not make much difference what the *mode of onset*, whether with *pneumonia*, pleurisy, laryngitis or hæmoptysis, if this class of symptoms are present, *Sulphur* must at least begin the remedial treatment. *Psorinum* is its most natural complementary. This is, of course, in cases that have passed the acute stage or affection. Not only here is *Sulphur* the remedy, but with the same symptoms in those *latent types*, where no marked recognizable ailment has preceded. The disease makes considerable progress before there are serious symptoms to arouse the patient, and it is remarkable how slight the lung symptoms may have been.

Tuberculinum or *Bacillinum* is indicated if there is a *family history of tuberculosis.* The patient complains that he *takes a fresh cold* ever little while, and he don't know how. *Loses flesh* even *while eating well.* Short dry hacking cough, < mornings when he may raise little. Menses do not appear when they should in young girls. The deposit or pain is like *Sulphur* often located in the *apex of the left lung*. There are ever changing symptoms, affecting first one organ, then another, travelling around like *Pulsatilla*, to lungs, skin, brain, kidneys, stomach, etc., and the pains like those of *Belladonna* come and go suddenly. Burnett in his little book on cure of consumption with the *Bacilli virus* is very convincing, and my own use of it is in several cases very gratifying. He used in his cases the "C," which I suppose means the 100th potency. I have used the 30th, 200th, 1 m. and C. M. with good effect; but the preparation that has given me the best results in several instances is the D. M., made on my own fluxion machine. I almost hesitate to make such a statement because of the prejudice in the minds of many, but believe it to be better to tell the truth whether it is accepted or not. The next remedy is

Calcarea ostrearum. The symptoms and indications leading to the choice of this remedy in incipient consumption, or first stage of the established disease, will be found as much, or in many cases even more, in the constitution and early history of the patient than in the local manifestations. Indeed no true homœopath will ever lose sight of this in any remedy. Homœopathy cannot be limited to the symptoms and pathological changes of a locality, but must take in the whole patient. If the history of the case is that of a *sweaty headed child*, with *tardy closing of the fontanelles*, *too much fat* and too *tardy or irregular bone developements*, and *delayed dentition; sweaty head* which soaks the pillow, and the leucophlegmatic constitution is still found in youth and adult age. If the boys are subject to *epistaxis*, the girls *menstruate too early*, and then too profusely until the climacteric; they are as cold and susceptible to cold, with feet and legs as cold as *Sulphur* is hot and burning, we will have an entirely different case from that of *Sulphur* to begin on. We might go on and give the whole list of characteristic symptoms of this remedy of wide range and deep action, but that would be *Materia*

Medica, where it can all be found. But we will notice here the local symptoms that lead to indicate this drug. *Painless hoarseness*, $<$ mornings, sensation of dust or feather down in larynx, trachea, lungs, causing tickling irritation to cough. The BREATH BECOMES SHORT, ESPECIALLY ON GOING UP STAIRS OR AN EMINENCE (*Arsen.*). Later on mucus rattles in the chest. The cough is at first dry, *especially* at night; and finally becomes loose, *especially in the morning*, when there may be profuse salty sputum. During the cough there may be *pain and rawness* (*Caust.*) in the chest. There is SORE PAIN IN THE CHEST AS IF BEATEN (*Arn.*), *the entire chest is painfully sensitive to touch* (*even extremely*) *and on inspiration. Calcarea* acts strongly on the *middle right lung*, but is not by any means confined there.

The expectoration differs in the different stages of the disease, in the first stage, white, gray, yellow, frothy or gluey; later becomes thicker and heavier, yellow. fetid; or gray-yellow of putrid odor. It becomes heavy and falls to the bottom, when spat into water with a "*trail of tough mucus behind like a falling star*."—Fellger.

"In young consumptives of a *Calcarea* diathesis where abscesses form, the pus having a fetid or putrid odor, after the pus is discharged, *Calcarea* in a high potency may effect a complete cure."—(Guernsey).

The next remedy of prime importance, and ranking as high as either of the preceding ones, is.

Phosphorus. A considerable "talk has been said" about this being a dangerous remedy to use. Farrington says "I would not advise you to give *Phosphorus* in well marked tuberculous patients If tubercles have been deposited in the lungs you should hesitate before giving it, unless the picture calling for it is so strong that you cannot possibly make a mistake." I think the "picture" should be strong for any remedy, and if not strong should be cause for hesitation. The greatest danger in giving a well indicated remedy in tuberculosis in any stage of the disease is in giving it too low or two frequently repeated. And this danger is not confined to *Phosphorus*. Rummel says only once in fifteen days. Dr. Charge, of Paris, confirms him. But the safest rule is not to repeat as long as improvement continues, and then in another potency. Now for a few "leaders." This remedy is generally found indicated in tall, slender, narrow chested persons, with fair, delicate skin, long silky eyelashes, highly sensitive organization; brilliant mental faculties but defective physical development.

Especially young persons who have grown too rapidly, incline to stoop in walking (like *Sulphur*), hollow chested and anæmic or chlorotic. There is often pronounced nervous debility; trembling; weakness and prostration. Hæmorrhagic tendency, vicarous, epistaxis, or even *small wounds bleed much.* Hæmorrhage of the lung is sometimes the first symptom. Takes cold easily and every cold inclines to settle on the chest, *Pneumonia* is easily contracted, and for its treatment, to save repetition, I will refer you to the article on that disease. These are the general indications.

The local are: Hoarseness. < in the evening (*Carbo. veg.*). Cannot talk, the larynx is so painful. Breathing short, oppressed, sense of heaviness in chest. Cough, *dry*, constant, from tickling in the throat-pit, with tightness or constriction across the upper third of chest; spasmodic, hollow, from tickling or irritation under sternum; hurts chest, holds it with hands for relief (*Bry.*, *Eupat. perf.*), severe, *shakes the whole body*; < *in cold air*, from laughing, talking or singing (*Spong.*), and especially *when lying on left side*, also apt to be < in evening until midnight (Raue). Expectoration scanty at first; in first stage; later, bloody, purulent, rust colored, salt, sour or sweet. Of course, there are many other symptoms that may be present, but these are leading ones, and when present the remedy properly exhibited as to dose and repetition is capable of great good, no matter at what stage of the disease.

Hepar sulphur, combining the properties of both *Sulphur* and *Calcarea ost.*, and also possessing those peculiar to the combination, must never be forgotten in the first stage of this disease. The *Hepar* patient is *extremely hypersensitive*, not only to pain, but to touch, even to the *exposure of any part of the body to cold.* He is always taking cold, in this resembling the *Tuberculinum.* The tendency to eruptions is like *Sulphur*, and they are inclined to be pustular or to form abscesses and are always *extremely sensitive to touch.* On the other hand, *Hepar* is like the *Calcarea* element, so sensitive to cold air, wants to be wrapped up even in warm weather (*Psorin.*). The nervous system is just as sensitive as is the skin. He is angry at the slightest cause, and *faints with the pains* if he has any. Great tendency to pus formations, whether in lungs or elsewhere; also to croupous membrane formations. So far as local manifestations are concerned the larynx and trachea are favorite points of attack in both children and adults, so that the tubercular deposit is particularly apt to light there at the first. It is one of our best remedies for laryngeal phthisis. As elsewhere, the larynx is *sensitive to cold air*, and to touch, croupy manifestations, and the child is, or was when young, always having croupy attacks from the least exposure, especially to cold, northwest winds. The

COUGH is dry, hoarse, or croupy sounding at first; but afterwards becomes loose, wheezing and rattling, and is < from *cold air* (even the exposure of a hand or foot) or uncovering; touching the parts (larynx or throat) or swallowing, especially solid foods (parts so sensitive). The BREATHING is wheezing, whistling, often asthmatic, must sit up and bend the head backward. If he can cough up the mucus with which the tubes seem loaded relief for a time follows. The SPUTUM varies from scanty, tenacious, muco-purulent, to pus-like, bloody, tuberculous masses, or small balls, which, when crushed, emit a carrion-like odor. But the leading characteristic is the exceeding hypersensitiveness, both mental and physical. No remedy can surpass it here, and it is capable of checking the progress of a tuberculosis if not too far along, and greatly ameliorating if too far advanced to hope for a radical cure.

Arsenicum alb. With this remedy the general condition of the patient leads more positively to its use than the local manifestations, though the indication of Dr. R. R. Gregg is a very reliable characteristic, as I myself have frequently proven, viz., *sharp, fixed or darting pain in apex and through upper third of the right lung.* In general the patient begins to grow weak or complains of great prostration, especially on attempting to exercise or ascend an eminence. An anæmic condition is common. Emaciation begins and the old school physician will now prescribe the inevitable cod-liver oil, to supply the waste, without removing the cause. The BREATHING is accelerated, rapid, oppressed and accompanied with restlessness and anxiety, all < by exertion and *lying down*, and especially at *midnight.* It is apt to become asthmatic at times, with much wheezing and constriction. The COUGH is < *on lying down* and on rising in the morning. It is also often < at *midnight* or *1 to 3 a. m.*, especially when the asthmatic symptoms are present. The EXPECTORATION is characteristically *frothy saliva.* Here it outranks all other remedies. Bloody sputum is often present and mixed with the froth. Many other symptoms may be present and confirm these. Cases coming from, or following the abuse of alcohol, tobacco and Quinine often find their remedy in *Arsenicum.*

Sanguinaria. I bring this remedy in here as one often adapted to the incipient stage of phthisis, because I have so often seen its good effects in such cases. It is particularly indicated in those cases supervening upon pneumonia or bronchitis, where the cough hangs on, at first dry and hacking, but later becomes very loose with profuse expectoration, which is VERY OFFENSIVE SMELLING even to the patient himself. The cheeks flush up with circumscribed redness, especially in the P. M., flushes of heat pass over the body, in head, chest, stomach or abdomen. The pain and sometimes soreness and fullness is most pronounced in the *right chest* and extends to the right shoulder, which it is often difficult to put into use to raise the hand to the head.

While I have put these remedies in first place as likely to be indicated in the first or incipient stage, I would not for a moment seek to leave the impression that *many times* other remedies must be preferred according to indications. Again while it is true that they are often adapted to this stage it must not be supposed that they may not be useful in any stage. Such an idea would lead to a lamentable routinism in the art of prescribing, and is the weak point in old school therapeutics.

I will now follow with a few leading indications of other remedies which are liable to be indicated in this stage. And I am more anxious to do this, realizing the importance of a good *beginning* in the treatment of this so intractable a complaint under the ordinary methods.

Bryonia. Jahr wrote in his Practice—"If the cough is quite dry I give to women *Bryonia*, and *Nux vomica* to men, according to circumstances." Ah! that last "*according to circumstances*" is the saving clause. Then he adds—In their case other remedies may be required, such as *Aconite*, *China*, *Ipecac.*, *Hepar*, *Spongia*, *Drosera*, according to the indications given in chapter XX, 2, 5–7. Turning to those chapters we find under Bronchitis, Laryngitis, Pneumonia, etc., a *great number* of remedies from which to make choice.

Jahr was a master and knew better than to rest his case on a few routine remedies. No more can we. *Bryonia* is one of the first remedies if as the exciting cause of an incipient tuberculosis in a patient predisposed thereto a Pneumonia, especially a pleuro-pneumonia, has been suffered. And it is on what are called pathological as well as symptomalogical indications that we may, or must, base our choice. The hepatized lung does not clear of the exudate, or the pleuritic effusion has been imperfectly absorbed, or not at all. Many forms of Phthisis commence in this way. If the proper remedial treatment is applied early we will not have these plastic exudates to deal with ; but many times we are called too late to do so. So we must do the best we can at the later stages.

The cough remains and may be still *dry* and *painful*, causing the patient to *hold the chest* with the hands. It *hurts the head* to cough, and is always, or nearly so, *worse on motion*, or coming in out *of cold air into a warm room*, or *after eating*, causing retching and vomiting. Stitching pains in chest are more pronounced during the acute pneumonia or pleuritis, but may still continue in a greater or less degree. The appetite is poor, but there is often much *thirst for large quantities* at long intervals, and the lips are *dry and parched* and sometimes cracked. This shows a lingering internal fever. Other symptoms and a number of them may be present for this so well known remedy. A knowledge of the pathogenesis of the drug will disclose them. The aggravations are < *on motion*; exertion; A. M.; hot weather; rising up from lying (gets faint); going from cold into warm room. Ameliorated by lying on the painful side; pressure; rest; perfect quiet; cold and eating cold things.

Pulsatilla. Is indicated in those cases of lung trouble which, instead of having a dry cough, the cough becomes loose, and the expectoration is of *yellow or green mucus*, with *bitter taste*, sometimes *streaked with blood.* The tongue is coated white, *with little or no thirst*, and loss of taste and sometimes smell, and the discharge from the nose corresponds with that expectorated. The menses have not appeared as they should; the patient grows weak, short breathed, especially oppressed in a *close warm room*, and feels much better in open air, though she chills easily, and if in pain *chilly* with the pains. This is a picture of a case following an acute attack of bronchial or lung trouble. But there is another phase that is of equal importance. It is when the patient has had a suppression of the menses. Especially by chilling or *wetting the feet*, or in young girls where they do not come on or are delayed. The patient becomes chlorotic, chilly, and has the same aggravation indoors as above, and is greatly relieved in open air, also unlike *Bryonia* is better when moving slowly around. She has erratic *pains*, now here, now there, and is generally very *sad* and *inclines much to weeping* over her condition. This state is of course found very often in the well known *Pulsatilla* temperament. These are a *few* of the *leading* symptoms and this remedy is almost sure to check the progress of an incipient consumption if wisely applied. Let me say right here, that if the patient is of a psoric constitution, *Sulphur*, of course, must not be forgotten, but if not that *Tuberculinum* high complements *Pulsatilla* as well as *Sulphur* does *Bryonia;* of course, according to indications which will often be found.

Alumina. Is another remedy that is very useful in chlorotic women, who are disposed to catarrhal discharges from mucous membranes. It is well adapted to the first stage of the disease and is best adapted to spare, dark-complexioned women. It is especially useful in cases weakened by a profuse leucorrhœa, who are greatly exhausted at the menstrual period, or when they should occur. The appetite is subject to vagaries, like longings for *starch*, *chalk*, rags, cloves, tea-grounds, etc., etc., as is often found in chlorotic. The patient gets hoarse, or may suffer from follicular pharyngitis, with elongated uvula. The breathing becomes short and oppressed, and the cough is generally dry and < in the morning, when she succeeds after long coughing in raising a little thin mucus. As a rule the remedy is chosen not so much by the local as by the general symptoms of the

Alumina patient. *Alumina* and *Bryonia* complement each other well, as would be expected from their corresponding symptoms and constitution; but the *Bryonia* is oftener adapted to the cases coming on after acute affection of the respiratory organs.

Causticum is a remedy of which the old school knows almost nothing, and it is not well understood by all who call themselves homœopaths.

It is of first importance in those cases where laryngeal trouble is the first symptom. There is great hoarseness, *worse in the morning, with rawness, burning and soreness in the chest.* Dry, hacking COUGH, with soreness in the chest and in a *streak down the trachea.* There is sometimes *involuntary spurting of urine* with the cough, cough is worse when *exhaling* and is relieved by a swallow of cold water. There is very little expectoration. It *cannot be raised* but *must be swallowed.* The hoarseness and inability to expectorate seems to be due to a weakness or semi-paralytic state, and general weakness and paralytic tendency seem to characterize this drug generally. *Soreness, rawness* and *burning* is found in all mucous membranes and especially in those of the respiratory tract. Psoric and sycotic manifestations are additional indications for the use of this remedy. It is often well followed by *Sulphur* or *Carbo veg.* This latter when the hoarseness changes from morning to evening. But we will have more to say of this latter remedy when we come to the second or more advanced stage of the disease.

China off. and *Ferrum* are remedies that are to be

considered in cases of pronounced anæmia, the former especially in those cases which have been brought there by *hæmorrhages* or other loss of fluids such as seminal or suppurative, etc., etc. In these cases we will find great weakness, anæmic headaches with ringing or noises in the head and ears; digestion is impaired; with *great flatulence*, and sometimes chronic diarrhœa, which is painless and accompanied with noisy flatus; exhausting sweats; everything, loss of blood, semen, pus, stools and sweat seem to combine to empty out the life of the patient. Another thing I have found very characteristic, viz., the patient is *worse every other day*. If this state is not met chest and lung symptoms will follow. Hoarseness, oppressed breathing, cough, all aggravated when the *head lies low*. The chest is extremely sensitive, cannot bear auscultation or percussion (like *Calcarea*); the cough is worse from deep inspiration (*Phos.*); talking (*Phos.*); laughing (*Phos.*); after eating (*Bry.*); light touch of the larynx (*Lach.*); least draught (*Hepar*); lying with head low (*Hyos.*, *Spongia*), etc., etc. The expectoration is of various kinds, nothing very characteristic. This remedy complements *Ferrum*, as would naturally be expected. *China* may be indicated in any stage of the disease, but is particularly useful to prevent the development of tubercles in cases exsanguined or greatly reduced by *loss of fluids*.

Ferrum is particularly useful in those cases of congestive anæmia, eristhitic chlorosis, or phthisis florida so common in young people, especially girls.

The old school stumbled upon that as they did upon the anti-malarial properties of Quinine, and knowing nothing of the law of similars and the small dose, better than the large one, accomplished much harm with both. It seems to me that nothing but the most pig-headed prejudice could have hindered an honest investigation of Hahnemann and his methods, which would have resulted in showing them when and how to use these agents wisely and well.

The subject for *Ferrum* is the *pale*, *chlorotic*, *weak*, *delicate woman*, *who easily flushes in the face on the least excitement.* There is great paleness of the lips and cavity of the mouth, in fact of the mucous membranes generally. The young of both sexes, notwithstanding the anæmic condition, are very prone to *local congestions* of a severe type. This is especially true of the chest, and there are pains *flying from one point to another*. *Blood spitting*, *epistaxis*, *profuse menstruation* is common. The breathing is oppressed as from orgasm of blood, and the expectoration is blood streaked; or hæmoptysis of bright blood interspersed with dark coagula like the profuse menses which it sometimes takes the place of, vicarous is often present. *Ferrum* is a *bleeder like China*, and the bleedings are the result of the local congestions aforementioned. (I want to here call attention to another remedy that is equally prone to such local congestions, viz., *Sulphur*, but with the latter remedy the lips and orifices are VERY RED instead of *very pale.*) The cough like that of *China* is varied, but the bloody expectoration is very apt to be in evidence.

The exploded theory that the anæmia is to be cured by Iron as a blood food is not to be considered, for if this element is deficient the fault lies in the assimilative processes, and must be corrected by the homœopathically indicated remedy, if at all. Out of this theory have come all the abuses of this truly valuable medicine. Hence, it follows that Iron like all other remedies must be given in the homœopathic form to get really *curative* results. *Ferrum* is especially useful for splenic troubles, which are almost always coupled with anæmic states, from the abuse of Quinine. Sometimes the entering wedge that opens the way for the ingress of the little microbic devil to gain a foothold, by weakening the *vital force*, so as to render it incapable of defending the citadel in which it rightfully resides, is some liver trouble. The pulmonary trouble is secondary, but nevertheless fatal, and as truly tuberculous as from other beginnings. Three remedies that deserve especial consideration here are *Mercurius*, *Chelidonium* and *Carduus marianus.*

Mercurius, in the first place, if the miasm syphilis, either recent or remote, is an element in the case. The most common mode of attack is in a pleuro-pneumonia, of right side, with sharp stitching *pains through lower right chest to back;* bilious symptoms such as pain and tenderness in the right hypochondria, < *lying on right side*, vomiting, jaundice, etc., etc. The peculiar and characteristic mouth symptoms, *moist*, *slimy*, *sticky*, *without thirst*, *swollen flabby* most leading of all, the *sticky*, *profuse sweat without relief.* Here no remedy can substitute it and, properly exhibited, most wonderful and gratifying results follow.

In my observation *Mercurius* does not do very much for tuberculous subjects after this stage, except as I said before, unless syphilis is in the case, but

Chelidonium is different and may accomplish much in both the early and later stages. The first symptom that generally appears is the well-known persistent *pain under the inner angle of the right shoulder-blade.* It has also a *deep seated pain through the whole right side of chest.* Again, stitches in right side of chest, oppression of right chest, soreness of lower ribs of right side, pain in right shoulder, etc., etc. It is as preëminently a right sided remedy as is *Lycopodium*, and they complement each other well. There is a great deal of

COUGH, sometimes dry and spasmodic, with painful contraction of the abdomen with every cough; at other times there is much expectoration, < in morning. A peculiar symptom is that there is at times forcible ejection of mucus, which *flies out of the mouth in small lumps* (*Badiag.*, *Kali carb.*). Now, if there are the liver symptoms, colorless stools or the alternate *yellow as gold* diarrhœa, dark yellow, bile laden urine, yellow skin and sclerotica, there is no mistake. *Chelidonium* is the remedy, and will probably cure the whole *patient.* The use of the remedy should be persisted in, for it is a long deep acting remedy. I do not mean by this that it should be given continuously, without intermission, but given until relief, and then stopped and left to act as long as improvement continues, to be repeated again, and generally in a different potency, as occasion requires. Other remedies may have to be interpolated, generally antipsoric, like *Sulphur* or *Lycopodium*, especially the latter, during the course of the treatment. I was a little surprised not to find *Chelidonium* noticed in "Gregg" by Allen on consumption, but think it must have been an oversight, as no one knows better than Allen the wonderful value of this remedy. My attention was first called to *Chelidonium* as a remedy for incipient consumption in a little work by "Hitchman." I have lost the book, but have used the remedy many times with success.

Carduus marianus is the third of the trio here mentioned. It acts somewhat like *Chelidonium*, removing congestion (chronic) of the liver and right lung, and I have used it very satisfactorily in some cases after *Chelidonium* had done a great deal but not quite finished the cure. I cannot give so clear cut indications for its use, but have been guided mainly by "Hering's Guiding Symptoms" for my indications. I will therefore refer my reader to the same source of information. The *Natrums*, especially

Natrum mur. and *sulph.*, are important remedies in those cases which from an impoverished or disorganized condition of the blood, lead to the anæmic or chlorotic state which so frequently predisposes to consumption. It is especially valuable in cases of old, intermittent fever, that has been abused with

Quinine. The patient's assimilation is so impaired that, *while he eats well, he still emaciates* all the time. There may be much thirst, and yet the bowels are constipated, with much rectal trouble, or the opposite; watery mucous discharges take place here as they do in all the mucous membranes. With the COUGH there is generally copious, transparent, watery or albuminous expectoration. This is a picture particularly in part at least of *Natrum mur.*, while

Natrum sulph. has some symptoms and conditions peculiar to itself. This is Grauvogl's great *hydrogenoid* remedy, *i. e.*, always worse in *wet rainy weather.* They always feel better on a dry day, whether hot or cold. This is the constitution in which gonorrhœa works most perniciously. It is also an anti-sycotic remedy. Grauvogl ranks it with *Thuja* in this place. These things must be understood and recognized in our treatment of tuberculosis or any other chronic disease, if we obtain the best results; any of the three miasms of Hahnemann (Psora, Syphilis or Sycosis) once engrafted on the human organism weakens and not only predisposes to other diseases, but must be met and controlled in as great measure as possible by appropriate medication. *Nat. sulph.* has some very strong local symptoms calling for its use.

1st. There is an asthmatic condition which is < in wet weather, with great rattling and expectoration.

2d. There is much pain in the chest on coughing, especially in the *lower left lung* (right, *Kali carb.*, *Merc.*, *Chelid.*); the patient springs up in bed and holds the chest with the hands.

3d. There is this painful soreness with the *loose cough* so different from *Bryonia*, which is with the dry one. Such cases as these are often wonderfully relieved and sometimes cured with this remedy.

Sepia is entitled to a large place in the *Sepia* type of woman, whose tendency to tubercular trouble finds encouragement in a weakened sexual system. *Persistent leucorrhœa with a heavy bearing down sensation in the uterus, as if everything would come out, coupled with a weak, gone sensation in the pit of the stomach*, is its chief characteristic. The face of the *Sepia* subject is pale-yellow, or with yellow spots on face, around the mouth, or *yellow saddle across the upper part of the face and nose.* Great weakness or *generally relaxed* condition corresponding to that of the uterus and appendages is common. There are frequent flashes of fever or heat, with weakness quite similar to *Sulphur*, and but for the uterine symptoms so pronounced it might be difficult to differentiate between them. There are different kinds of *cough*, two of which are characteristic. One the patient coughs a dry persistent cough with gagging until a little mucus is raised, sometimes vomited, followed by relief; the other loose, OFFENSIVE, EXCESSIVELY FŒTID. It may be blood streaked, and tastes *salty*. *Sepia* is especially useful in women at the climacteric.

Iodine is one of our so-called anti-scrofulous remedies. A low cachectic condition with profound debility and great emaciation is generally present. The weakness like that of *Calcarea* is especially evident in the loss of breath on going up stairs, or *ascending an eminence*. *Arsenicum* also has this symptom strongly, but the *Calcarea* and *Arsenicum* constitution and temperament are quite different as a rule. *Iodine* is intensely *brunette;* dark eyes, complexion and hair; no remedy more so. The glands swell while the other tissues waste, sometimes the mammæ dwindle, but swell and are sore at the menses. Menses profuse, even cancerous disorganizations, or chronic leucorrhœa, which is profuse and so corrosive that it eats holes in the linen; but the most prominent symptom of all is—"ravenous hunger," wants to eat all the time, and loses flesh, too; is *greatly relieved by eating*, *always feels the best during*, *or immediately after*, *eating*. Most remarkable cures have been made with this medicine on these indications, as leaders to the remedy.

Nitric acid. In cases in which syphilis, or mercurialization, have brought the patient into a condition of susceptibility to consumption, which might never have occurred except for such a cause. Such cases occur and this remedy is indispensable. One of the first symptoms appearing is a *pricking in the throat as from splinters.* These prickings or sliver-like pains may be found elsewhere, as in chest, rectum, anus, etc., and are as characteristic as are the stinging pains of *Apis.* Affections of mucous outlets of body are common, as cracked corners of mouth, fissured rectum, vagina or bladder, flushes of heat in localities, or general (like *Sulphur*). Great general weakness and tendency to sweats at night. Bowels tend to looseness (chronic diarrhœa) instead of constipation, etc. These are the general symptoms which are leading, and the patient is like *Iodine* oftener than otherwise of the brunette type with rigid fibre, dark complexion, black hair and eyes. The local symptoms are not so characteristic as under some other remedies; but hoarseness, cough dry or loose, shortness of breath are commonly present, and especially the stitching or sticking pains (like splinters) are much in evidence *in the chest*, as elsewhere. *Bryonia* and *Kali carb.* are sometimes used for them when *Nitric acid* would do better. Dunham gave as characteristic *sticking pains in rectum when coughing; extremely strong and offensive urine* (smelling like horse urine).

Drosera and *Spongia* are especially to be remembered in laryngeal cases. They with *Hepar sulph.* and *Causticum* (already considered) form a quartette of which the homœopathist may well be proud. The old school do not know their great value. With *Drosera* there is hoarseness, voice hoarse, deep, requires exertion to speak, only able to speak in a *deep bass voice.* Tickling in the larynx causing cough, hurts so that the patient supports the larynx on coughing or swallowing. Soft, hard or green expectoration. Laryngeal phthisis, with hoarseness and emaciation. Deep sounding, trumpet-toned cough (*Verbascum*). Sometimes spasmodic with retraction of the muscles of the abdomen; must hold on with the hands. The cough is $<$ by lying down, laughing, singing, talking and after midnight. There may be stitching in the chest when sneezing or coughing, like *Bryonia*. The most characteristic symptoms are the *deep bass sound of voice and cough*, and the *constriction* of the muscles of the chest and abdomen. *Drosera* is particularly useful in those cases of consumption, which come on after *measles*.

Spongia has also great hoarseness. The cough is croupy in character. Everything seems perfectly dry and tight. There is difficulty in speaking, the voice is hollow, and gives out when singing or talking, and the larynx is sensitive to touch (*Lach.*). There is often *burning* in the larynx. Eating and drinking warm things relieves. The three

Kalis, viz., *bichromicum*, *carbonicum* and *iodatum*, have each of them very strong characteristics and may be indicated in any stage of the disease. The chief characteristic of the first is the *ropy*, *stringy discharge from all the mucous membranes, especially the expectoration.* It will hang down in long strings from the mouth to the floor. The remedy that comes nearest to it and is to be remembered, especially in bronchial consumption of the aged, is *Hydrastis Canadensis.* In *Kali bichromicum* cases there are almost always the prominent nose symptoms (see catarrh) present in greater or less degree. *Pains from back to sternum or sternum to back*, or sharp pain through apex of left lung (*Myrtus*, *Therid.*, *Pix liq.*, *Sulph.*). Cough is < 2 to 3 A. M. and when undressing (*Hep.*). Hoarseness < *in the evening*.

Kali carb. may be indicated in the first or incipient stage when after pleurisy or pneumonia there remains a *pain or soreness in the right lower lobe*, the pain may be dull or stitching in character. This remedy comes in particularly well after *Bryonia*, if that remedy did not remove all the trouble. No two remedies oftener complement *Bryonia* in such cases than *Sulphur* and *Kali carb.* The stitching pains of *Bryonia* are relieved by rest and pressure or lying on the affected side. But with *Kali carb.* the pains are not so relieved, and occur in different parts as well as in the chest. Other remedies having marked action on lower right chest are *Merc.* and *Chelid.* (*Nat. sulph.*—left). The COUGH is at first dry, hard and fatiguing, and characteristically < at 3 or 4 A. M. Later it becomes loose with much expectoration. These are a few only of the symptoms that may appear in a *Kali carb.* case. It is certainly a great remedy. *Kali carb.* and *Carbo veg.* complement each other well, of course only when indicated.

Kali iod. is no less important, and will often finish cases of acute bronchitis or pneumonia which would run the patient into consumption if not remedied. When there remains an obstinate cough after an acute bronchial or lung trouble, and there is profuse expectoration from low down, deep in the chest, as if it came from mid-sternum, with pain through to between the shoulders, and there are drenching, exhausting night sweats and weakness, there is no remedy better. In such cases there are two remedies that may compete with it, viz., *Sanguinaria* and *Stannum*. In all three the expectoration is profuse and thick, but in *Stannum* the matter tastes *sweet*, in *Sanguinaria* the matter is *fœtid* and *offensive*, even to the patient himself (*Sepia* and *Psorin.*), while with *Kali hyd.* it is *salty* (*Sep.*). With *Kali hyd.* and *Stannum* the expectoration is thick green, which is not so with *Sanguinaria*.

Sometimes with the *Kali hyd.* there is a frothy or soapsuds-like appearance of the sputa, but the *heavy*, *green*, *salty* expectoration is more characteristic. The frothy expectoration is found in œdema of the lungs and may occur in Bright's disease. One of the most astonishing and conclusive proofs of the dynamic power of drugs as developed by Hahnemann's process of trituration and dilution with percussion is

Carbo vegetabilis. It, like the *Kalis*, may be indicated in any stage of phthisis. If it begins in the larynx *with painless hoarseness; great roughness with deep rough voice* (*Dros.*) *which failed on exerting it;* < from damp evening air (*Caust.*, < mornings), this is the first remedy. It is particularly good for this condition in elderly people of broken down constitutions, venous system preponderating. But its use is by no means confined to the aged. The *Carbo veg.* subject is one of generally reduced vitality, which may or may not have followed on the heels of some acute disease from which she never recovered, is apt to be pale, anæmic, with scorbutic gums and flatulent and easily deranged stomach; much gas which presses upward (*Lyc.*, downward, intestinal) and is quite subject to hæmorrhages from gums, nose or lungs. A characteristic of these hæmorrhages with this remedy is the great *paleness of the skin*. The breathing is short, oppressed, wants more oxygen, *hunger for oxygen*, wants to be *fanned hard*, or has doors and windows open. Circulation is weak, with coldness of extremities, especially *knees*. There is sensation of weakness and fatigue in the chest, sometimes with *burning as from glowing coals*. Aching through *apex to right scapula* (left, *Myrtus*, *Sulph.*). It has two kinds of cough, one dry, hard, spasmodic, the other loose, with purulent, salty (*Kali hyd.*) or offensive sputa (*Sang.* and *Creosot.*). These with more symptoms show how valuable this remedy is. It is not used so often as it might be with great advantage, especially by the materialists who can see nothing above the twelfth potency. This and other remedies like *Nat mur.*, *Sepia*, etc., cannot be known in half their possibilities, and especially this one.

Lycopodium. This remedy, relegated by the old school to *baby land* (powder) because they do not and cannot know, as we do, the virtues of medicinal substances until they are willing to divest themselves of their prejudice, so far as to resort to our methods of proving drugs, is one of which we sing loud praises. So far as tubercular trouble is concerned it may be of use not only in pulmonary tuberculosis but in that kind of manifestation in any part or tissue. Again, it may be indicated in any stage of phthisis. In weak, puny, sickly bodies, with well developed heads, but irritable nervous people, who are peevish and cross, *especially after sleep;* persons of dark complexion (*Iod* and *Nit. ac*), intellectually keen, but weak and deficient in muscular development; upper part of body wasted, lower part semi-dropsical, with tubercular history or predisposed to lung or hepatic disease. This is the constitution and temperament that is most apt to develop *Lycop.* symptoms. It is one of the main remedies in which, as Professor Bennet says, the disease seems to begin as one of essentially faulty nutrition, for notwithstanding the emaciation, or tendency thereto, there is *canine hunger*, the more he eats the more he wants to; but in eating, while he feels as though he could eat a *ton*, the *first few mouthfuls fill him right up full*, and he can eat but little after all, or, on the other hand, there may be a *constant sense of satiety*, and excessive accumulation of flatulency, with much rumbling and gurgling in the intestines. These cases are often subjects of the lithic diathesis and often present red sand in clear watery urine, which may be accompanied with much pain in the region of the kidneys. All this may be controlled and the development of tuberculosis prevented by a skillful administration of *Lycopodium*.

Then again it is one of our very valuable remedies in advanced cases of tuberculosis. A badly treated or neglected pneumonia, where pneumonic infiltration or hepatization is remaining, and needs something to promote absorption, often finds help here in *Lycopodium*. Cough may be dry, or loose as if the chest were full of mucus, with rattling, and the expectoration thick, green, salty, or offensive. If there is fever (hectic) it is often worse from 4 to 8 P. M., and is *especial* indication for this remedy. I have seen even incurable, far advanced cases so improve as to astonish all observers.

It is wonderful the wide range of usefulness of this remedy when well chosen, and here let me say from long observation that the low or crude preparations of this drug are almost worthless. It must be used in the potencies from the 30th upward to get its best curative power.

Silicea is another remedy which, like *Calcarea* and *Lycopodium*, cures cases the result of mal-assimilation, and change the whole being of its subject from a sickly to a healthy and strong person. Of course, this is most easily and quickly done in youth and childhood. The best time to begin the treatment of tuberculosis is before they get it, or in scientific parlance, *prophylactic*. Rosenbaum writes (page 261 Physician versus Bacteriologist) thus: "In the interest of prognosis and therapy not only is the determination of the species of micro-organism present to a certain degree essential, but information as well regarding the *extent of irritability* to foreign bodies and their product (predisposition)." * * * "The demonstration of the microbes is of particular value only in this connection, the presence of tubercle bacilli in the sputum proves a certain *inferiority of the pulmonary tissue*, which condition prognosticates further changes of tissue and also creates the soil for the pyogenic organisms." To this "*inferiority*" of not only pulmonary but any tissue, homœopathy particularly addresses itself, and aims to render untenable the human organism as a "*soil*" adapted to the destructive organisms bacterial, etc. The physician who is able to recognize early the manifestations of a disordered *vital force*, and set it to rights, is far more efficient as a healer than those who are never able to act until the pathological or microbic appearances confirm a diagnosis. In other words, the anticipatory or prophylactic treatment, hygenic and remedial, is of paramount importance. So far as remedies are concerned, the homœopathist is able to meet the demand in his "*symptom correspondence*" treatment of the *patient* even before pathological lesions are "to the front" better than any other. This we claim, and it is "up to us" to be able in our knowledge of *Sulphur*, *Calcarea*, *Lycopod.*, *Psorinum*, *Tuberculinum* and the long list of well proven drugs to be able to choose wisely, and apply skillfully to this kind of patients. What are the leading symptoms pointing to *Silicea?* We give a few especially adapted to those who suffer from imperfect nourishment, not from defects in quality, or quantity, of food, but from *defective assimilation.*

Lean, emaciated body with weak ankles.

Disproportionately large head, which sweats.

Feels very sensitive to cold; lack of vital warmth, and is especially averse to uncovering of the head, > with it wrapped up.

Foot sweat which is offensive, and if checked brings on much suffering generally.

Yielding mind, discouraged, tearful (chronic of *Pulsatilla*), "grit all gone."

Tendency to suppurations, and glandular swellings.

Constipation, stool slips back when partially expelled, or persistent diarrhœa with changeable stools.

This is a picture of *Silicea*, which may be found in subjects tending to the development of tuberculosis and may check it. It also has its uses in the late stage of the disease, especially when the expectoration becomes *purulent* or muco-purulent, and may afford much comfort and lengthen life by controlling the suppurative process here as in other tissues, and modifying the night cough which is so fatiguing and weakening.

Kreosote used so indiscriminately, as it has been by the old school, on the microbe killing theory, has been of infinitely more harm than good. It has its place like other homœopathic remedies, and must, like the rest of them, be chosen according to indications. It is especially adapted to women who are of the hæmorrhagic type, who menstruate profusely and have corrosive, profuse leucorrhœas, with tendency to cancerous disorganizations. It is also especially useful where the expectoration is *copious*, *purulent*, *greenish-yellow or pus-like, and very offensive.* There are, of course, other indications for its use, but it is far from being a general panacea, such as the allopathists seek to make of it.

We have now gone over nearly forty of our leading remedies, and tried to give those indications for their use which, according to our observations, are leading and reliable. Of course, every one acquainted with the genius of Homœopathy well knows that we are liable often to have to seek our similimum outside these, but I am quite certain we will much oftener find our remedy among these.

The complications liable to arise, in the course of this disease (tuberculosis), are so many and various that we will not undertake to enumerate them. If an acute attack of bronchitis, pneumonia or pleurisy should arise the treatment would be found under those diseases. Of course, always taking into consideration the general tuberculous condition, which would make the treatment of the acute affection in some cases to vary from that of cases non-tuberculous.

Hæmoptysis, which is so often met in these cases, needs perhaps especial mention. Here, as elsewhere, the indicated remedy is the best styptic.

Ipecac is indicated when the hæmorrhage is profuse, comes up easily, or is vomited, blood bright red, preceded by a *sense of bubbling* in the chest. Cough with spitting of blood on the least effort. *Nausea* and wheezing or rattling in the chest.

Hamamelis. *Profuse hæmorrhage of venous blood;* comes into the mouth without any effort like a warm current.

Ferrum. Hæmorrhage in connection with the other *Ferrum* symptoms given under that remedy. Bleeding with pain flying around the chest, or *between the shoulders*, blood *bright-red*, anæmic persons or those who flush fiery red in the face by spells.

China, when the hæmorrhage is very profuse with fainting and *ringing in the ears* from loss of blood. Especially for the weakness following great loss of blood or other fluids.

Aconite, if there is great restlessness and *fearfulness*.

Carbo veg., if there is dark or light colored hæmorrhage with perfect indifference, especially if there is excessive paleness of the skin of whole body.

Opium, especially in drunkards, and if there is frothy appearance of the blood.

Many other remedies might be mentioned here, as they are in the books, and as hæmorrhage is only one out of many symptoms the choice must be made in accordance with the whole of the case. Auxilliary measures for the time being, put the patient in half reclining position, and enjoin perfect quiet. Give plenty of fresh air. Ligate upper left arm and thigh or both thighs and arms if necessary, when bleeding ceases gradually loosen ligatures. Hot water bag over cervical spine. If much blood has been lost, injections of normal salt solutions. Alcohol, Ergot and astringents do no good and may do harm (Gatchell).

Now a few words as to GENERAL MEASURES, which are all important.

Climatology is of first importance, dry air; high air (altitude); warm air (moderatley); pure air, out of door air. Colorado and New Mexico and the tablelands in Mexico stand first. For summer, the Adirondacks; for winter, West Virginia, East Tennessee, North Carolina, western part; Northern Georgia. The western slopes of the base of the Rocky Mountains from Colorado south is the best in this country and probably in the world. The altitude should be from 3,000 to 5,000 feet high. Even higher will work all right, except in people with weak heart. Change of altitude should not be made suddenly, especially in advanced cases. In case of improvement from change of climate and altitude, the patient should not return to low altitude or cold climate until cure or recovery is complete. Two mistakes are very common, viz.—*Going too late*, and *returning too soon*.

The directions for LUNG-DEVELOPMENT as given by Dr. Gatchell in his "Pocket Book" are as good as any. We quote: "The patient must take regular and systematic exercise in lung-developement and chest expansion.

"*Mèthod:* Practice (a) *abdominal* and (b) costal breathing.

"*Abdominal*—With all clothing perfectly free, lie upon the back on a firm, level surface; expel the air from the lungs, and depress the epigastrium to its extreme limit; then fill the lungs, causing the epigastrium to rise, making as great an excursion as possible. Repeat this ten times. Exercise in this way several times daily. *Costal breathing*:—The best way to develop the upper part of the chest is by exercises with two rings suspended from the ceiling by ropes. They should be on pulleys so as to be adjusted to different heights.

"(A). With the rings on a level with the shoulders, let the patient grasp the rings with the hands; with the feet fixed, lean far forward, extending the arms outward backward, *at the same time gradually inflating the lungs as the motion is made*. As the body is drawn back to the erect position, *expel the air from the lungs*. Repeat this many times.

"(B). Raise the rings above the head. Slowly draw

up the body on tip-toe, and let it down again, inhaling and exhaling as the two motions are made.

"(C). Many times daily, when in the open air, go through with this exercise: Place the hands on the hips, the fingers forward and thumbs backward; stand erect, and throw the shoulders and elbows well back; inflate the lungs fully, beginning by abdominal expansion and extending to the upper chest; close the glottis, hold for a moment. While holding the air in the lungs, make forcible effort at retraction of the abdominal muscles, pressing the diaphragm upwards. Then suddenly and forcibly expel the air (this last as regards the *forcible* expulsion need, modifying. It must not be too forcibly or violently expelled in very advanced cases for fear of rupturing vessels or causing soreness or inflammation, etc.). Do this many times daily. Continue all these exercises for years after recovery."

No exercise should be pushed to the point of great fatigue. Rest in open air should be enjoined after such exercise.

FEEDING. No iron clad rules can bind us here. "What is one man's meat is another's poison," holds good here as well as in health.

Super-alimentation must not be so super as to derange the stomach. This is the tendency. So far as cod liver oil is concerned it seems to agree well with some, not at all with others. Cream and milk with graham bread, especially if the patient is inclined to constipation, is very good in many cases. I like it better than cod liver oil. Meats may be varied, but the fats mixed in with mutton or beef is better than pork fat. Thompson's rules for feeding are perhaps as good as any. Alcoholics are especially to be avoided. The old "rock and rye" treatment so loudly recommended by whiskey drinkers or sellers has killed many a patient that might have recovered under other means. With those who are not able to avail themselves of the benefits of change of air, altitude, climate, etc., let them make a point of what is called "out of door" treatment. Room where the sun shines in during the day, windows open night and day or no windows at all in, and bed clothing enough to protect against weather exposure, is all important.

I have not seen medicine taken by inhalation do any good, but for moral effect and introducing plenty of air into the lungs some inert substance may be used, if you cannot satisfy the patient otherwise. All these things as to general measures are well and helpful, but the "*main chance*" is in the skillful application of the *Similimum*.

COUGH.

Cough, as we have often been informed, is but a *symptom*, and occurs in many diseases. Its importance as a guide to the similimum, when taken as to the kind of cough, whether dry or loose; by what aggravated or ameliorated, and its accompaniments or concomitants, is well known to the true homœopath. Therefore, although there is a repertory attached to this work which should be consulted as to single characteristic symptoms, we have concluded to give a list here of prominent cough remedies in such a way as to lead, if possible, more directly to the remedy than by the circuitous route of the whole Materia Medica. In this case we will begin in the usual way with

ACONITE.

Character—Generally *dry*, short, clear, ringing, whistling, or *croupy*.

Excited, or < in the evening; at night, during *expiration;* dry cold winds or currents of air; deep inspiration; smoking or drinking.

Ameliorated by nothing marked.

Accompanied by *short breath*, *stitching pains*, *fever*, *restlessness and agonized tossing about*.

In a general way *Aconite* is mostly indicated in the first stage of all acute inflammatory diseases of the respiratory organs. But unless the concomitant symptoms, especially FEARFUL *restlessness*, and agonized tossing about, as well as high temperature and rapid pulse are present, the *Belladonna* or some other remedy having equally intense inflammatory symptoms may have to be preferred.

ANTIMONIUM TART.

Character—Predominantly loose, with *coarse rattling of mucus*, which is often difficult or impossible to raise. Bronchia and chest seem loaded with it. Seems as though a cupful would be expectorated with each cough, but little comes up.

Aggravation—< as the accumulation increases and when lying down.

Amelioration—> on expectoration and on sitting up

Accompanied by—Yawning, *dozing and sleepiness;* cyanosis from carbonized air; twitching; short breath from suppressed expectoration; coarse rattling of mucus; hepatization.

This condition calling for *Antimon. tart.* may be found in la grippe, pneumonia, broncho-pneumonia, bronchiectasis, senile catarrh, capillary bronchitis of children, œdema of the lungs, atalectasis, emphysema and threatened paralysis of the lungs. It is especially found useful at both ends of life (children and old age), though by no means confined there. It resembles most perhaps *Ipecac* (in children), but the noises (in *Ipec.*) from the mucus in the tubes is more of an asthmatic or wheezing nature. In the later stage of broncho-pneumatic troubles when the cyanotic state, and the *coarse rattling* mucus does not yield to *Tartar em.*, *Carbo veg*. follows well after it, and *Sulphur* or *Lycopod.* later, to finish cure the case.

BELLADONNA.

Character—Short, dry, tearing, spasmodic, hoarse; generally little or no expectoration.

Excited by—*dryness*, *scraping*, tickling or *burning* in the larynx.

Aggravated by—< evening and night, most violent after midnight; talking or crying; deep inspiration and when awaking.

Ameliorated—Eating or drinking warm things.

Accompaniments—Crying before cough; *red*, *injected sore throat;* redness of the eyes; tightness or congested chest; congestion to head and chest with high fever, quick pulse, throbbing carotids, headache, often delirium.

Belladonna like *Aconite* is oftenest found useful in the first stage of acute inflammatory affections of the respiratory organs. *Aconite* oftener in croup; *Belladonna* in bronchitis; *Aconite* in pleuritis; *Belladonna* in congestion of the lungs; *Aconite* with great excitement and *fearful* anguish; *Belladonna* with semi-stupor, strong head symptoms and delirium; *twitching* in sleep, or spasms. *Aconite* dry, hot skin, no sweat and does not want to be covered. *Belladonna* wants to be covered and *sweats* on *covered* parts. They follow each other well, but should not be alternated or combined, and will not be by a GOOD prescriber. Although so useful in acute diseases, they may often be called for in acute aggravations often arising during the course of chronic.

BRYONIA ALBA.

Character—Predominantly *dry*, but in pneumonia sputa tough and hard to separate, falling in a jelly-like lump, light in color, or of a soft brick shade.

Aggravated by—< *motion; eating or drinking; coming from cold air into warm room;* on breathing deeply.

Ameliorated by—> *perfect quiet; pressing hand upon chest; lying on painful side.*

Concomitants—*Stitches in chest; pain in head as if it would burst; pain and soreness in chest, must support it with hand when coughing. Constant disposition to expand the chest or sigh deeply.* Short breath < on motion; pleuritic stitches < on motion and inspiration; effusions into the pleural cavity; stitching pains in region of heart; *generally < on motion.*

In acute inflammations of the respiratory organs *Bryonia* is not so often indicated in the first or congestive stage as *Aconite*, *Belladonna* or *Ferrum phos.*, but rather in the second stage when effusion, hepatization or the *products* of inflammation are appearing. Then it becomes the prime remedy if the *symptoms* characterizing the drug appear. In coughs which persist after the inflammatory stage is past, or in which this stage was not very pronounced, it is still one of our best remedies. Cough < by coming from cold air into warm room is characteristic (*Nat. carb.*), and the soreness of the chest also (*Caust.*, *Eupat.*

perf. and *Nat. sul.*). Stitches in chest finds a remedy not only in *Bryonia*, but in *Kali carb.* and *Squills.* The *Kali carb.* stitches occur any time and are not necessarily < on motion like those of *Bryonia.* In a general way the *thirst*, *dry mouth and lips* and dry, hard constipation, as well as < of all symptoms on *motion* are all corroboratory for *Bryonia.*

CALCAREA CARB.

Character—*Dry at night ;* loose A. M. and day with yellowish expectoration, sometimes salty, sweetish, putrid ; excited by sense of plug or dust in larynx. Expectoration sinks in water with a trail of tough mucus behind, like a falling star (Felger).

Aggravation—< damp, cold air, raw, damp winds, wet weather, washing or working in cold water ; ascending, talking, morning ; and evening after midnight ; mental excitement.

Amelioration—> dry warm air, after breakfast, lying on painful side.

Concomitants—*Hoarseness < mornings ;* SHORTNESS OF BREATH ; < ON SLIGHTEST ASCENT ; SORE PAIN IN CHEST AS IF BEATEN, *painfully sensitive to touch and inspiration ;* acts more on middle and upper right lobe. Infra-clavicular depression ; LEUCOPHLEGMATIC CONSTITUTION.

This is one of our greatest remedies for tuberculosis. For a comparison of this and *Sulphur*, ranking equally with it, especially in the incipient stage, I must refer you to my Leaders in Hom. Therapeutics. It would require too much space here. It is perhaps well here to emphasize the peculiar temperament (*Leucophlegmatic*) in which it is most useful. Of course it may become very useful in other than purely this temperament, but it will be the exception and not the rule. This difference between *Calcarea* and *Sulphur* may be noted that the former may often be indicated in any stage of the disease, *Sulph.* not so frequently, but the "symptoms" and "personnel" must decide even in the exceptional cases. The potencies will do very much better than the low or crude drug. Not often indicated in acute respiratory troubles.

CARBO VEG.

Character—Dry, spasmodic, continuous (in whooping cough), or, expectorates *purulent matter* as in tuberculosis.

Excited by—Itching in the larynx or roughness or crawling in the throat.

Aggravated by—< evening or midnight ; going from warm to cold places ; damp air.

Concomitants—*Hoarseness* and *rawness* < *evenings* or *damp air;* breathing short ; *wants to be fanned; burning* in the chest ; hæmoptysis, with *pale cold skin; weak*, *fatigued* feeling in the chest ; pneumonia, *fetid sputum*, cold breath and sweat, rattling breathing, threatened paralysis, cold knees, etc.

See remarks under *Antimonium tart.* Many cases of pneumonia that have seemed hopeless, in a state of collapse, blood stagnating in the capillaries, causing blueness, coldness and ecchymosis, with the foregoing chest symptoms, may be saved by this remedy. The difference between *Carbo veg.* and *Arsenicum* in this stage is that the erethism and restlessness is very marked under the latter, and lack of manifestation of vital force under the *Carbo veg.* It is not only here in these affections that *Carbo veg.* is useful, but in typhoids and other diseases where these conditions are present.

CAUSTICUM.

Character—Mostly dry, sometimes mucus, which it is difficult to raise; must swallow it; hollow racking cough.

Aggravated—< *by bending forward*; from *exhaling*.

Ameliorated—> *by a swallow of cold water.*

Accompaniments—Sensation as if patient could not cough deep enough to raise mucus; *soreness in chest as if raw; tightness of chest*, wants to take a deep breath; *pain in hip; involuntary escape of urine; hoarseness with rawness in throat and chest;* worse MORNINGS; cannot speak aloud, muscles refuse to act; influenza with tired sensation in limbs and rheumatic pains.

One of our best remedies for cough, following after colds, the *hoarseness*, *soreness* and involuntary escape of urine being leading symptoms. The *soreness in the chest* may be compared with *Bryonia*, *Eupatorium*, *Nux vomica* and *Natrum sulphuricum.* The *Bryonia* often has pains in the head and is always < on movement. In *Eupatorium* the bone-pains are greatest. The *Natrum sulph.*, unlike either, generally has *loose* cough with the soreness, and often a pain in left lower chest. *Causticum* is often attended with greater weakness, almost semi-paralytic. *Arnica* and *Phosphorus* must also be remembered in cough with soreness of the chest, both having peculiar symptoms accompanying by which to differentiate.

CHAMOMILLA.

Character—Scraping dry cough, caused by *tickling in pit of throat;* < at *night without waking*, especially after taking cold in children. The child becomes angry, then coughs. Winter coughs; coughs all winter.

Aggravation—< winter, from cold in sleep.

Ameliorated—> getting warm in bed.

Concomitants—Hoarseness with rawness and scraping in the larynx. *Tickling in throat pit.* Suppression of measles. High fever with hot sweat about the head, and one red hot cheek and the other pale and cold.

This remedy is found oftenest indicated in children when there is great nervousness. The child is ugly, cries for apparently nothing, is cross and ugly, and will not be quiet unless *carried.* In temper it comes nearest to *Cina*, but with *Cina* the face flushes up with *circumscribed redness* in paroxysms, and presents the class of so-called worm symptoms so common in children. It (*Cham.*) is especially useful if the child is teething, with the many nervous symptoms common to such irritation, such as sleepiness, twitching, even spasms, with weeping, howling and tossing about. Nervous, hysterical women who anger easily also come in its range, with similar nervous symptoms.

CINA.

Character—Generally dry; spasmodic, or continual hacking; paroxysmal.

Excited or caused by helminthiasis.

Aggravated—< at night, or fretting, drinking, walking in open air; pressing on larynx; when awaking from sleep.

Ameliorated—> sometimes at night.

Concomitants—*Gagging*, spasms, twitching, unconsciousness, rattling, vomiting; rubbing the nose, paleness around mouth and nose; alternate canine hunger and loss of appetite, restlessness and screaming in sleep, flashes of intense fever with intensly circumscribed red cheeks.

All this, as is well known, is a picture of helminthiasis, which will complicate and aggravate almost every form of disease in children. It is not necessary; it is not best to give this drug in its alkaloid to *expel* the worms, but will do much better in the potencies. Yet I have found as I have with other alkaloids, such as Quinine and Strychnia, that when the *Cinchona*, *Nux vomica* or *Cina* seemed indicated and did not work satisfactorily, the alkaloid would. I do not know why. One thing must be guarded against, viz., prescribing the remedy for "worrums" regardless of indications. I knew an intractable case of rheumatism which resisted *Bryonia*, which seemed indicated, which was promptly cured by *Cina*, which has symptoms similar to the *Bryonia*.

DROSERA.

Character—Deep sounding (*Verbasc.*) hoarse cough; spasmodic cough, with great constriction in chest and hypochondria, so that the patient has to support these parts with his hands; spasmodic cough with retching and vomiting.

Aggravated—< by warmth; drinking, tobacco smoke; laughing; singing; weeping after lying down, *after midnight* or in the morning.

Concomitants—Low, hoarse, deep *bass voice;* constriction of the larynx; sensation as of a *feather in larynx*, constant tickling, preventing sleep.

This remedy with *Ipecac* and *Cuprum* form a trio of remedies for spasmodic coughs similar to whooping cough, which is very valuable, and we might add *Cina* to make a quartette. *Drosera* and *Cuprum* are equally spasmodic, *Ipecac* has more mucus and asthmatic wheezing, and *Cina* the so-called worm symptoms. I do not find great difficulty in choosing between them.

But *Drosera* is also a great remedy for chronic or acute laryngeal troubles, and the choice may here be between it and *Hepar sulph.* and *Causticum.* All have great hoarseness, but the deep bass voice stands strongest under *Drosera.* Laryngeal or even pulmonary phthisis may be warded off or cured by these remedies if not too far along.

DULCAMARA.

Character—Cough may be dry and hoarse, or *loose with much mucus.*

Caused—by exposure to *damp*, *cold* air, such air *suddenly following warm air.*

Aggravated—< by deep inspiration; lying down, or warm room.

Ameliorated—> out of doors.

Concomitants—Much mucus in the chest, which is *difficult to raise;* mucous rales.

Dulcamara is prone to spend its action with mucous membranes generally, and especially on the respiratory organs. So-called *catarrhal affections*, especially in the first stage, coming on after exposure to *damp cold*, are amenable to its curative action. Its action on the skin is almost equally marked, and suppressed sweat or skin eruptions and these catarrhal states often alternate and find a valuable remedy in *Dulcamara*. *Dulcamara* being so susceptible to sudden changes from dry warm to damp cold makes it especially useful in mountainous regions in vacation time, when the days are warm and nights cool. Also near the sea shore where these varieties of weather so suddenly alternate. Equable temperature is not the place for *Dulcamara*.

HEPAR SULPH.

Character—Dry and hoarse; at other times LOOSE

and RATTLING; chocking; wheezing; croupy; paroxysmal.

Caused by—Exposure to cold, especially to *dry, cold air*, west or northwest winds.

Aggravated—< *when slightest portion of body becomes uncovered*, limb getting cold; eating or drinking anything cold; *towards morning;* after eating.

Ameliorated—> *wrapping up; keeping warm.*

Concomitants—Hoarseness < in cold air; croup or bronchitis, with *wheezing and rattling of mucus*, difficult to expectorate; soreness and weakness in chest; pneumonia or abscess of lungs; pleurisy with croupous exudates; consumption.

A combination of the two great polychrests, *Sulphur* and *Calcarea carb.*, still developing those belonging to neither alone, this becomes one of our greatest polychrests. The action toward catarrhal affections of the membranes, even to the degree of croupy formations, and suppurative destruction, is not found so strongly in any remedy. Again the exceeding sensitiveness to pain, touch and mental irritability, *even to fainting*, is most prominent. This exceeding sensitiveness is especially manifest in the suffering caused by the *least exposure to cold air. China* and *Silicea* must be remembered here. *Ulcers and eruptions are sensitive to touch.* Everywhere and all the time *sensitiveness.* While the cough symptoms are well defined these constitutional symptoms are always found associated. No remedy will better repay a careful and thorough study to understand its genius.

HYOSCYAMUS.

Character—Dry, hacking, persistent, spasmodic cough ; little or no expectoration.

Aggravation—< *when lying down.*

Amelioration—> *when, sitting up.*

Concomitants—Stupor or furious delirium ; mucous râles in typhoid pneumonia.

Not a remedy of wide range in respiratory troubles, but so positive in its sphere that it becomes invaluable.

In typhoid pneumonia and scarlatina it stands close to *Rhus toxicod.*, but the delirium or stupor is greater and will do more in those cases than the *Rhus.* If *Hyoscyamus* had no other use than here it would be indispensable. But it does the cough so markedly, < on lying and > on sitting up is often found in catarrhal colds, and even in well gone cases of consumption. In fact, in any case of this kind it must be remembered. Again it is particularly useful for the same cough in *old people.*

IGNATIA.

Character—Dry, persistent, continual. Rarely any expectoration.

Aggravated—< *by coughing.* The more she coughs the more she wants to. The longer the cough the more the irritation to cough, < when he stands still. < warm drink.

Ameliorated—> by walking, or diverting the mind.

Concomitants—Sleepy after the coughing spell,

Sighing, or wants to take a long breath. Spasmodic contraction of the chest. Especially useful in nervous or hysterical people.

This is one of the symptoms of the paradoxes of this remedy, viz., the irritation to cough increases with coughing. It is in keeping with the roaring in the ears > by music; piles > by walking; sore throat > when swallowing; empty feeling in stomach not > by eating, etc. It is the remedy of contradictions, such as is often found in nervous, hysterical persons. There is another place where I have found *Ignatia* to be excellent—that is, in the persistent cough following some cases of grippe. The patient can't get rid of that irritable and persistent cough, though she otherwise improves. *Ignatia* 1000th, B. and T., cures such cases like magic. Try it.

IPECAC.

Character—Sometimes *dry*, at others *loose*. Spasmodic often.

Aggravation—< motion, and open air.

Amelioration—> warmth, and quiet.

Concomitants—*Fine rattling or rather wheezing in bronchial tubes, from large accumulation of mucus. Violent dyspnœa, with wheezing; accumulation of mucus threatens to suffocate; loses breath with the cough, turns pale and stiffens; nausea, retching, or vomiting with cough; whooping cough with nosebleed; blue face; rigidity during paroxysm; phlegm rattling everywhere on chest; hæmorrhage profuse, bright red.*

Any one who can interpret symptoms can see how useful this remedy might become in asthma, whooping cough or catarrhal pneumonia of children. And so it is, and especially so if the persistent *nausea* so characteristic of the remedy is present. The wheezing breathing may find a similar remedy in *Arsenicum* and *Cuprum*. If the mucus becomes looser and with coarse rattling, we would prefer *Antimonium tart.*, *China*, *Dulcam.*, *Kali sulph.*, *Lycopod.* or *Pulsatilla* or *Carbo veg.*, and each one has symptoms enabling us to choose. There is not room here to differentiate. It is very interesting and entertaining for each physician to do this for himself, and thus, after practice, which makes perfect, become an expert in the art of prescribing.

KALI BICHROM.

Character—Dry, with tickling in the throat, or loose with great accumulation of mucus. *Hoarse, croupy.*

Aggravation—< evening or toward morning (*Hep.*), < *2 to 3 a. m.;* after eating or drinking; *when undressing.*

Amelioration—> lying down or getting warm in bed.

Concomitants—*Pain from mid-sternum to back. Expectorations glutinous, stringy. Croupy exudations in the larynx and bronchi.* Membranous croup, bronchitis, phthisis pulmonalis, etc. It is equally efficacious in the chronic or acute forms. *Pain through apex of left lung to shoulder.*

The leading indication is the tenacious, stringy mucus which hangs down to the floor in a ropy string, and it is found in all the mucous membranes as well as the respiratory. In fact, it leads all remedies for this. *Hydrastis Canadensis* and *Lyssin* approach it most nearly. *Coccus cacti* must also be remembered here, especially in whooping cough. For the formations of membranes *Bromine*, *Iodine* and *Hepar sulph.* stand along side, but none of them have the peculiar stringy expectoration. In stomach trouble, where the same stringy mucus is found under *Kali bich.*, *Iris versicolor* is to be preferred if the characteristic *burning* of the membranes is present.

KALI CARBONICA.

Character—Dry, hard, exhausting; sometimes *with purulent expectorations*, mixed with blood and thin mucus; or white *masses fly* from the mouth (*Badiaga*).

Aggravation—< *warm food*, *exercise*, lying *on left side; 3 a. m. all* symptoms.

Amelioration—> *after breakfast.*

Accompaniments—*Stitching pains everywhere, but especially in right lower chest through to back. Sac like swelling of upper eyelids. Chilliness at noon*, *at night heat*, *weakness of the chest.* Much inclined to take cold (*Tuberc.*). Adapted especially to anæmic or dropsical constitutions.

This remedy, of which Hahnemann said "persons suffering from ulcerations of the lungs can scarcely get well without this antipsoric," is certainly one of our very best. The location of the pain, *lower right chest*, is very valuable. *Mercury* and *Chelidon.* also act here, while *Sanguinaria* and *Calcarea* act on the middle lobe, same side. *Arsenicum*, upper right to back. Upper left, *Therid.*, *Anis.*, *Pix liquida*, *Sulph.* and *Tuberculin.*, etc., of course other indications agreeing. The *stitching* pains occur everywhere. Even temples, eyes, teeth, etc., but are not necessarily < and by motion as are those of *Bryonia*, except in pleurisy where they may be. Suppressed or delayed menses in young women, with much pain and weakness in the back, may be saved from consumption by this remedy.

KALI IOD.

Character—Suffocative cough, later with *copious green sputa*, or *frothy like soap-suds.*

Concomitants—*Stitches through sternum to back, or deep in the chest, < walking; purulent sputum; exhausting night sweats; rapid emaciation; great weakness.* In persons who have been mercurialized or of a scrofulous diathesis.

These cases often run into phthisis pulmonalis. They generally begin as a hard cold, and end in pneumonia, or bronchitis, and "hang fire" in convalescence. Two other remedies should be also remembered here, viz., *Sanguinaria* and *Stannum.* In all three the expectoration is profuse and thick, but in *Stannum* the matter tastes sweet, while in *Sanguinaria* the sputa are very *fetid*, offensive to the patient himself (also *Sepia* and *Psorin.*). *Kali iod.*

is *salty* tasting (*Sep.*). *Carbo veg.* has green expectorationsometimes, as does also *Lycopod.*, but with the latter it is often *grayish* and salty, and with *Pulsatilla* the taste is often *bitter* like the mouth and taste generally.

LACHESIS.

Character—Generally *dry*, but if any expectoration, it is *scanty*, and difficult to raise, but > follows raising. Violent and long continued.

Aggravation—< *falling asleep; after sleep;* in sleep *without waking* (*Cham.*).

Amelioration—> after *raising a little.*

Concomitants—Larynx *painful to touch*, or *bending head back.* Don't want anything to touch throat or chest. Acts most intensely on the left side generally. Fever < *p. m.* Stools *offensive.* Disturbed circulation as at the climacteric. Cardiac complications.

No remedy is more positive in its sphere. Whether in croup, laryngitis, bronchitis or pneumonia, the foregoing symptoms guiding, we are almost sure of benefit. Sometimes the choice will fall upon *Naja*, especially in coughs coupled with heart troubles, and we have a strong team in the two. *Aggravation from constriction* is its general and almost invariable chief modality and is found almost everywhere. It is the opposite of *Bryonia* in this particular which is relieved by pressure. Perhaps the nearest relative to *Lachesis* in the matter of constriction is *Cactus grand.*, which has a distressing *sense of constriction* which is also found in many parts. It is well to remember the two remedies together, especially in heart affections.

LYCOPODIUM.

Character—Dry, day and night, fatiguing, or loose in the morning with *grayish yellow, salty sputum.*

Aggravations—< *4 to 8 p. m.;* on *alternate days; stretching out the arms; stooping or lying;* in a *warm room.*

Concomitants—Chilly *4 to 8 p. m.; feet cold, 7 p. m. Flushes of heat towards evening,* vomiting sour between chill and heat; thirst for small quantities during fever (*Ars.*). *Sweats easily;* wants to uncover. *Affects right side* most, or goes from there to the left. Unresolved pneumonias, especially with liver complications. *Much flatulence.* Red sand in the urine.

Lycopodium is a remedy of wide range, and deep action. It should never be given below the 12th potency as its remedial properties are not developed below that. Raue verified it in "a case with expectoration of large quantities of pus, cough day and night, hectic fever, circumscribed redness of the cheeks." Others have done the same. Many of the symptoms indicating *Lycopodium* in respiratory diseases often lie outside the local trouble, such as the stomach, liver and abdominal. This is what distinguishes homœopathy from old schoolism, that regards as paramount the local pathology of the case. *Tuberculinum* is often a valuable complementary, or can be interpolated with advantage in cases having a tubercular history.

MERCURIUS.

Character—*Racking cough*, in the evening or at *night*.

Aggravations—Night air; dampness.

Concomitants—*Creeping chilliness in evening*. Chill *with heat of face*. *Fluent coryza*, in epidemic form. Sore throat, with *salivation*, *bad breath*, *flabby tongue with indented edges;* all this followed by *bronchitic inflammation or pneumonic or pleuro-pneumonic trouble, with pains in lower right chest to back; can't lie on right side; heat and profuse sweat which does not relieve.*

Bryonia has often been used for pneumonic or pleuritic affections when *Mercury* would have done better, but there are marked differences. *Bryonia* is better lying on the affected side. *Merc.* <, especially if it is on the right side or with liver complication. *Bryonia* mouth is dry with thirst. *Mercury* is moist and slimy with equal thirst. Sweat relieves with *Bryonia*, and aggravates with *Mercury*, etc. Some alternate these two remedies, but it is better to differentiate and give them singly. *Mercury* is seldom of much use in chronic respiratory affections, but in acute stands equally with *Aconite*, *Belladonna* and *Bryonia*, and its indications are well pronounced.

NUX VOMICA.

Character—Dry fatiguing cough, seldom loose.

Aggravations—< after eating or drinking; mental

or physical exertion; when lying on the back; when cold; *early in the morning.*

Ameliorated—> in *warmth* or when quiet.

Concomitants—*Hoarseness with roughness* or sense of *rawness in the nose and throat* < *inspiring cold air.* Chilliness on the *least motion*, even when peevish. Pain in *head or abdomen* on coughing. Generally sensitive, irritable and ugly. Specially in literary subjects who lead a sedentary life.

This remedy like *Mercurius* is seldom of much use in chronic respiratory trouble, only as it may be called for in dietetic errors and sufferings therefrom. But it is often the best remedy in the acute stages of common colds, especially if *Aconite* or *Bryonia* have only half cured the case. It follows well, *i. e.*, of course if indicated by the *symptoms.* The pain in head on coughing is found strong under *Nux vom.*, *Bryonia*, *Lycopod.* and *Capsicum.* The nervous constitution and disposition of *Nux vom.* are so *patent* that its success in our hands has led to its abuse (as usual) in the form of its alkaloid in old school hands. They never know when to stop with *enough.*

PHOSPHORUS.

Character — *Dry tickling cough; hollow cough; harsh, irritating cough; loose cough, with muco-purulent expectoration.*

Aggravation—< *when entering a room; or going from warm into cold air;* from odors; before a thunder storm; *evening till midnight;* laughing, talking, eating, drinking; *lying on left side.*

Amelioration—> *after sleeping; lying on right side; from cold drink;* pressure on chest.

Accompaniments — *Tightness across chest;* burning soreness, *pain in larynx* (aching); splitting headache; *night sweats, burning in back between shoulders.* Thin, light haired, slender people, inclined to cough. Flat chested, short breathed.

Many more symptoms, both objective and subjective, might be added, but these are *leading.* The rest of the picture must be found in the Materia Medica, as must those of all the other remedies. In acute inflammations of the respiratory organs, as well as in chronic, this is one of the most valuable of remedies. See pneumonia for its especial sphere of action there. Also tuberculosis for indications there. *Phosphorus* and *Bryonia* come quite close together, yet there are generally diagnostic points that are quite reliable. They follow each other well, as do also *Sulphur* and *Phosphorus. Rumex* is another remedy that should come into the list for comparison and *Causticum* must not be left out. *Bryonia, Phosphorus, Sulph., Causticum, Rumex,* quintette.

PULSATILLA.

Character—*Dry cough* at night or evening, after lying down. *Loose cough* with copious expectoration of *bitter* or tasteless mucus; < on lying down.

Aggravation—< *evening; on lying down.*

Amelioration—> sitting up; and cool air.

Accompaniment—Second stage of catarrhal colds with thick discharge from nose which is *bland* in character. Throat sore, raw, with *distended veins.* Aphonia, can't speak loud. Loss of taste, or bitter taste. *Constant chilliness*, but generally *aggravated in warm room*, with oppressed breathing. Phlegmatic subjects. Mild, yielding, tearful, inclined to despondency; easily moved to tears.

The respiratory troubles of *Pulsatilla* are often connected with menstrual irregularities, chilling or wetting the feet, especially when menstruating, or in amenorrhœa. Again in the sequelæ of measles, where hoarseness and loose cough follows and obstinately persists. This is where those who have any tendency to lung trouble are often set going in that direction. In the loose rattling cough with other *Pulsatilla* symptoms a timely and judicious use of this remedy may avert consumption. *Kali sulphuricum* is its chronic and may be found to be a "finisher" in obstinate cases. *Pulsatilla*, *Stannum*, *Kali hydroid.*, *Sepia* and *Sulphur* form another quintette to be studied in such cases.

PSORINUM.

Character—Dry cough, provoked by a *tickling* in the larynx or trachea, or loose cough of GREEN MUCUS, nearly like matter. *Winter cough.*

Aggravated—< in evening; on lying down.

Ameliorated—> keeping quiet.

Concomitants—*Takes cold easily*, *feels as though took cold every little exposure.* *Sensitiveness to cold air* or change of weather; wears a fur cap in the summer. Especially adapted to the psoric constitution, which is prone to eruptions. *Body has a filthy smell* even after bathing. All excretions offensive. Mind awfully depressed.

A nosode, but well proven, as all nosodes should be, and clinical verifications in abundance. *Medorrhinum*, *Syphilinum*, *Anti-toxine*, *Tuoerculin* and many other disease products are fast coming to the front as indispensable curative agencies. *Sulphur* and *Psorinum* stand very near together, but have characteristics that are positive. Both are powerful antipsorics. The red, raw orifices that characterize so strongly *Sulphur* are not prominent under *Psorinum*. Neither are the universally offensive excretions of *Psorinum* found under *Sulphur*. There are many other marked differences which a study will show. Notwithstanding they follow each other well, supplementing what the other could not do, an understanding of both will be a great advantage.

RUMEX.

Character—*Dry*, *incessant*, *fatiguing*.

Aggravation—< changing room; evening and night; touching or pressing throat pit; *slightest inhalation of cold air;* covers the mouth with the bed clothes.

Amelioration—> *warm air*.

Concomitants—*Tickling in throat pit; tickling in supra-sternal fossa; soreness behind sternum;* infra clavicular pain; stitching, stinging pain through left lung. Night cough of phthisis;

morning diarrhœa; itching eruption, < when undressing in cold air.

A remedy of not very wide range, but wonderfully efficacious within it. It compares with *Causticum* in its sensation of *rawness* along the tract, and with *Phosphorus* in its aggravation or inspiration of cold air. With *Chamomilla* in the *tickling* in the throat-pit, and with *Therid.*, *Anisum*, *Pix liquida*, *Sulph.* and *Tuberculinum* in the pain in left upper chest. Again it must be remembered with *Sulphur* for the morning diarrhœa, and with *Oleander*, *Hepar sul.* and *Nat. sul.* for the skin trouble. I have found it especially useful in the 30th, though many use it lower and some much higher with apparently equal success.

SANGUINARIA.

Character—Cough dry, excited by tickling in *larynx* or *stomach*, or crawling sensation behind sternum. Cough compelling *erect posture*, ceasing on passing flatus *up* or *down*. Loose cough with sputa *smelling very offensive*, even to the patient.

Accompaniments—*Pain in right middle chest. Burning in chest. Flushes of heat* over body with *circumscribed redness of cheeks*, *soreness*, *burning and smarting*. In persons subject to sick headaches. Pain (rheumatic) in right shoulder and arm.

This remedy may be called for in desperate cases of *pneumonia*, and here the circumscribed redness of the cheeks, one or both, is prominent. It follows *Phosphorus* well. The burning heat and flushings ally it with *Phosphorus* and *Sulphur*. It is especially useful when a *pneumonia* or acute bronchitis runs into a chronic form, the cough gets loose with copious and offensive expectoration and consumption is to be feared. It has done magnificent work here. The choice will often lie between it and *Kali hyd.*, *Stannum* and *Carbo veg*. Of course, the symptoms must here, as elsewhere, decide between them.

SENEGA.

Character—Cough dry at first, later *much mucus with wheezing and oppression.*

Aggravation—< evening and night, during rest, lying (on left side), on *walking* fast.

Concomitants—*Soreness in chest walls* remaining after an attack of bronchitis. Bronchial catarrh, or asthma with great accumulation of mucus, especially in the aged. Muscles of the chest and pleura involved; exudations in the pleura or hydrothorax.

The severe and persistent cough and oppression of breath as a consequence of the great accumulation of mucus is the most characteristic indication for *Senega*. I have relieved several cases of the worst asthma I have ever seen with this remedy. It will help when *Ipecac*, *Arsenicum* and *Lobelia* are powerless. It is a great remedy in coughs, not generally appreciated by the profession. I have never found it of any use in these affections in the potencies. Five or six drops in a glass of water, given in tablespoonful doses, one to two hours apart, then at longer intervals as improvement sets in.

SILICEA.

Character—Dry at first, later loose and *purulent*, or *muco-purulent.* Sometimes *musty* or fetid.

Aggravation—< *cold drink*, *motion*, speaking, *lying down*, *night cough.*

Concomitants—Pain in the chest; *weakness* in the chest (*Stann.*); difficult to *speak; shortness of breath*, < *exercise*, *lying on the back*, *want of animal heat*, *always chilly; sense of hair on the tongue;* night sweats, most after midnight; weakened or difficult assimilation; eats enough but does not nourish; foot sweats, or consequence of its suppression; *generally better in warmth, especially covering head.*

It will be seen that it is in chronic coughs that *Silicea* is most apt to be needed, the constitutional symptoms guiding to the choice even more than the cough. As elsewhere the tendency to suppurations or cavities in the lungs is an important factor. Here it may be between *Silicea* and *Kali carb.*, or if there is profuse discharge greatly weakening the patient—*China. Calcarea hypophos.* has a wonderful influence over suppurative processes, as I have had occasion to witness, but my experience is that it must be given low but carefully, as it sometimes excites hemorrhage, while on the contrary *Silicea* must be given high, and sometimes *very* high, to get the best results. The 6oooth acts beautifully.

SPONGIA.

Character—Dry, hoarse, barking, like a saw driven through a board.

Aggravation—< in evening, *talking*, *singing*, *laughing*, hot room or lying.

Ameliorated—> eating or drinking, *especially warm things*.

Concomitants—*Great hoarseness with soreness and burning in the larynx;* larynx sensitive to touch; breathing, wheezing, anxious < inhalation; blood seems to rush to chest; dyspnœa, > *bending forward*, < lying down; goitre. Acts on apex of left lung. Acts best on blondes.

Reference to our article on croup or laryngitis will further define its sphere. It is best known in this disease where its efficacy is unquestioned, but it is also very useful in the first stage of bronchitis and pneumonia. A cardiac cough where the patient awakens suddenly out of sleep with great suffocation, alarm and anxiety is often wonderfully relieved by this remedy even in incurable valvular disease, and I have several times observed the bellows sound of long standing consequent on acute inflammatory rheumatism entirely disappear after its use in the 1,000th potency (B. & T.). In laryngeal affections it ranks with *Iodine*, *Bromine*, *Kali bichromicum*, *Causticum*, *Drosera* and *Verbascum*.

STANNUM.

Character—The most characteristic cough of *Stannum* is LOOSE. Expectoration *thick*, *yellow or green*. SWEET or saltish (*Kali hyd.* or *Sepia*).

Aggravations—*Singing*, laughing, lying on *right side* (left side, *Phos.*).

Concomitants—Empty WEAKNESS IN STERNAL region. Great *general exhaustion* or *weakness;* can hardly talk loud on account of the *weakness in the chest.* All the weakness seems to center there. Sweats *night* or *morning*, most on *back.*

Several remedies have the sense of *weakness* in the chest, such as *Carbo veg.*, *Phos. acid*, *Spongia* and *Sulphur.* The *Carbo veg.* is < in the morning on washing; *Spongia* after *walking; Phos. acid* in young people who are growing too fast, or in onanists. *Sulphur* in the peculiar *Sulphur* subjects of psoric tendencies. Expectoration thick green, comes also under *Pulsatilla* and *Kali iodatum.* This is one of the remedies which certainly disproves the theory that the metals cannot be dissolved so as to be potentized, for I have seen the most positive and convincing cures made with this remedy in the 500th (B. & T.), and even much higher. So also with *Ferrum*, *Gold*, *Platina* and *Zinc.* Theory and prejudice must stand "from under."

SULPHUR.

Character—*Dry*, *short*, *violent.* Dry cough, *worse nights*, at other times loose cough, with *rattling* and *gagging;* expectoration greenish lumps, or sometimes blood mixed *with pus.* Sputa oppressive (*Psor.* and *Sang.*).

Aggravation—< talking, eating, *breathing in cold air*, lying.

Amelioration—> sitting up.

Concomitants—Chest sensitive on percussion, in

spots. *Soreness or stitch in upper portion of left chest. Burning in chest* with *heat in face.* Rattling *in chest when talking; weakness* in *chest. Flushes of heat all over. Burning in feet. Faint spells. Want of air, wants window open.*

This remedy has such a wide range of action and covers so many symptoms that it is apt to come into use in many cases, and especially if on account of psoric complications other seemingly indicated remedies do not act. It will become, as Hering used to call it, a "finisher" of acute cases which convalesce unsatisfactorily. It promotes absorption of disease products, as effusions, etc., and promotes the resolution of unresolved pneumonias, the hepatizations, etc. It will cover many cases of incipient phthisis, and here *must* be given *high* to get its best work. No remedy has a wider range of action, or deeper and more lasting results. It is especially indispensable in chronic diseases and in those tending to become so.

TUBERCULINUM.

Character—All kinds of cough. In the first stage *dry.* Later *loose, very loose,* with profuse expectoration.

Modalities not well marked.

Concomitants—Takes *cold after cold,* don't know how, but in every breath of fresh air. *Emaciation rapid and pronounced.* Symptoms *changeable,* especially pains changing, *now here, now there.* Tubercular deposit in apex of lungs; *oftenest left.*

Notwithstanding the prejudice against nosodes, we are forced to admit that they are wonderful remedies in certain cases. Clinical results not only with *Tuberculin* and *Psorinum*, as well as the others, cannot be ignored. Von Behring suspects that *Antitoxine* as well as *Variolin* acts along homœopathic lines, and is man enough to *say* so, and declares that if honest investigation takes him along homœopathic lines he goes that way. When this spirit takes possession of the old school in general the medical millennium is not far away. More honest investigation of this remedy will define its exact place as clearly as that of *Psorinum.*

Now that we have finished the arrangement of over thirty of our leading cough remedies we will be satisfied to give a few leading characteristics of those that are not so prominent, but are still of great value when indicated:

Acalypha.—Cough with expectoration of bright blood in *the morning, dark in the evening.*

Allium cepa.—Cough which so hurts the larynx that the patient grasps at it.

Alumina.—Every morning a long attack of dry cough, ending with slight expectoration.

Ammonium carb.—Cough at 3 or 4 a. m.

Ambra grisea.—Violent spasmodic cough, with frequent *eructations,* especially old women.

Aralia racemosa.—Spasmodic cough at night, *awakens after first sleep;* asthma.

Arnica.—Cough with soreness of chest; cries before the cough, *fears the hurt.*

Arsenicum alb.—Cough with asthma worse 1 to 3 a. m. Suffocating, must sit up.

Badiaga.—Paroxysms of spasmodic cough; *viscid mucus flies out of the mouth; cough causes sneezing.*

Baryta.—Cough connected with swollen tonsils.

Borax.—Expectoration smells *mouldy.*

Capsicum.—Cough expels an offensive breath from the lungs; cough hurts the head, *grasps the head with the hands.*

Chelidonium.—Cough with pain in chest *under right shoulder-blade.* Deep cough with expectoration.

Coccus cacti.—Cough with expectoration of much *viscid albuminous mucus*, draws out in long strings.

Coffea.—Spasmodic, or dry hacking cough, especially *after or during meals.*

Conium.—Cough from dry spot in the larynx, < *on first lying down.*

Corallium.—Violent, spasmodic cough, the coughs occur in rapid succession. "Minute gun" cough all day.

Cuprum.—Very violent spasmodic cough, with constriction of chest which almost shuts off breathing.

Copaiva.—Chronic pulmonary catarrh with profuse expectoration.

Eupatorium perf.—Rough scraping cough, chest sore, must support it with the hands.

Guaiacum.—Extremely offensive expectoration in phthisis.

Hamamelis.—Cough with varicose condition of the throat.

Hydrastis.—Senile catarrh; *thick*, *yellow*, *tenacious stringy sputa.*

Laurocerasus.—Continuous cough at night, from *heart disease;* cannot lie down.

Lobelia inflata.—Cough with *asthmatic constriction* of the air tubes.

Manganum.—Cough > on *lying down.*

Naja trip.—Irritative cough sympathetic with heart disease (weak heart).

Natrum carb.—Cough on entering warm room (*Bry.*), coldness between scapula (*Am. mur.*).

Natrum mur.—*Cough, with bursting pain in forehead.*

Natrum sulph.—Loose cough with great *soreness* in the chest, > from springing up and *holding chest with hands.*

Opium.—*Cough of drunkards*, dry or with frothy, bloody expectoration.

Phellandrium.—Last stage of consumption, where the expectoration is horribly offensive.

Phos. acid.—Cough in onanists, with expectoration of herbaceous smell (*Borax*), and weak chest.

Rhus tox.—Dry teasing cough, with *taste of blood.*

Sambucus.—*Sudden nocturnal suffocative attacks of cough*, wheezing crowing breathing.

Scilla.—Loose cough, morning expectoration with weakness, < or brought on by a drink of cold water.

Sticta pulm.—Incessant, wearing racking cough in consumptives, dryness of nasal mucous membranes.

Verbascum.—Deep, hollow, trumpet-toned cough.

Zinc. met.—Cough with such as have large varices; < after eating sweet things and *before and during the menses.*

Kali sulph.—Much *rattling of mucus* in the chest.

PREFACE TO REPERTORY.

All abbreviated remedies in this repertory preceded by the figure (1) are of first importance such as would appear in capitals or black-faced type in the various repertories. All preceded by the figure (2) are not quite so strong, but are the same as the verified or italicized type in the repertories. There are not one of either class but have been *verified.*

REPERTORY

LARYNX AND TRACHEA.

Catarrh: (1) Merc., Ars., Nux-v., All-c., Hep., Kali-bi., Nat-m.; (2) ant-t., calc., sul.; *sudden:* (1) Ars. LARYNX: (1) Rumx.; (2) calc., calc-p., calc-s. TRACHEA: (1) Rumx.

Constriction: (2) bell., cocc., ip. LARYNX: (1) Phos.; (2) bell., brom., dros., ign., mosch., nux-v.; *cough, during:* (2) ars.; *singing agg.:* (1) Agar.; *sleeping, while:* (2) lach., spong.; *after:* (2) lach., phos.; *talking, while:* (2) dros. TRACHEA: (1) Ars.; (2) brom., lach., phos., spong.; *evening, lying down, on:* (2) ars.

Crawling, LARYNX: (1) Con.; (2) caps., carb-v., caust., dros., thuj.; *sitting, while:* (2) psor. TRACHEA: (2) caps.

Croup: (1) Acon., Spong., Hep., Brom., Kali-bi., Lach., Phos.; (2) ant-t., ars., bell., cham., sang.; *exposure to cold dry air, after:* (1) Acon., Hep.; *gangrenous:* (2) ars.; *membranous:* (1) Kali-bi., Brom., Phos., Iod., Lach.; (2) apis, hep., kali-chl., sang.; *recurrent:* (2) calc., phos.; *sleep, after, agg.:* (1) Lach.; *extending to trachea:* (1) Kali-bi.; (2) iod., kali-chl., phos.

Dryness, LARYNX: (1) Bell., Con., Lach.; (2) caust., dros., phos., spong.; *aversion to drink:* (1) Bell. TRACHEA: (2) acon., carb-v., iod., lyc., spong.; *close room:* (2) puls.

Dust, *as from:* (1) Ars., Calc., Dros.; (2) chin., ign., puls.

Flapping *sensation,* LARYNX: (2) lach.

Flesh *hanging in* LARYNX, *sensation of:* (2) phos.

Foreign *substance,* LARYNX: (2) arg-m., dros., phos.

Inflammation, LARYNX: (1) Acon., All-c., Dros., Gels.; (2) arg-m., lach.. rumx.; *singers, in:* (1) Arg-n., Arg-m.; *speakers, of:* (1) Arum-t.; (2) carb-v.; *syphilitic:* (2) hep., iod., merc., nit-ac. TRACHEA: (2) acon., brom., hep., rumx., sang., spong.

Itching, LARYNX: (2) arg-n.; *night:* (2) cist.; *cough, from:* (2) carb-v., nux-v. TRACHEA: (1) Puls.; (2) ambr., cist., nux-v.

Laryngismus, *stridulus:* (1) Gels., Mosch., Ign., Bell., (2) iod., lach., meph., samb., spong.; *night:* (2) samb.; *midnight waking out of sound sleep:* (2) samb.; *expiration, on:* (2) chel., chlor.; *swallowing agg.:* (2) cupr.

Mucus *in air passages:* (1) Kali-bi.; (2) ars., cupr., seneg., stann. LARYNX; (1) Kali-bi.; *morning:* (1) Nat-m.; (2) kali-bi.; *blue:* (2) kali-bi.; *green:* (2) hep.; *tenacious:* (1) Kali-bi.; *tough:* (1) Kali-bi.; *transparent:* (2) nat-m. TRACHEA: (1) Arum-t., Squill., Stann.; (2) dulc., seneg.; *forenoon:* (1) Stann.

Œdema, *glottidis:* (1) Apis, Kali-bi.; (2) crot-h., lach.; *vocal cords:* (1) Lach.

Pain, LARYNX: (1) All-c., Phos., Lach.; (2) arum-t., calc., iod., kali-bi.; *blowing nose, on:* (2) caust.; *coughing, on:* (2) all-c., brom., carb-v., caust., lach., phos., spong.; *grasps the larynx:* (1) All-c.; *torn loose, as if something were being:* (1) All-c.; (2) calc.; *pressure, on:* (1) Phos.; (2) ars.; *singing, when:* (1) Spong.; (2) acon.; *speaking, after:* (1) Phos.; (2) acon.; *swallowing, on:* (1) Spong.; *talking, while:* (1) Phos., Spong.; (2) acon., bell.; *touch, on:* (2) ant-t., spong. TRACHEA, *coughing, on:* (1) Bry., Kali-bi., Caust., Phos.; (2) rumx., sang.; *in a streak down;* (1) Caust. BURNING: (1) Cact.; (2) am-m., ars., carb-v., spong.; *cough, during:* (2) spong. LARYNX: (1) Acon., Nit-ac.; (2) ars., bell., canth., phos., spong. TRACHEA: (2) caust., iod., merc-c., spong. CUTTING, LARYNX, *coughing, on:* (1) All-c. RAWNESS *in air passages:* (2) arg-m., carb-v., caust., coc-c., phos.; *coughing, from:* (2) coc-c. LARYNX: (1) Arg-m., Cham., Lach., Phos.; (2) caust., hydr., kali-i., sul.; *evening:* (1) Phos.; *clearing the throat, when:* (2) carb-v.; *coughing, from:* (1) Arg-m., Brom., Puls., Sul.; (2) arg-n., caust., rumex. TRACHEA: (1) Arg-m., Phos., Rumex; (2) caust.; *coughing, when:* (2) arg-n.; *talking:* (1) Arg-m. SORENESS: (1) Carb-v., Phos., Stann., Sul.; (2) arg-m., caust. LARYNX: (1) Dros., Spong.; (2) arg-m., brom., caust., kali-bi., phos.; *morning:* (2) arg-m.; *coughing, on:* (2) arg-m., brom., dros., phos.; *swallowing, on:* (1) Dros.; *touch:* (1) Acon., Spong., Phos.; (2) caust. TRACHEA: (1) Rumex; (2) caust., phos.; *coughing, on:* (1) Caust., Stann.; (2) arg-n. STINGING, LARYNX: (1) Nit-ac. STITCH-

ING, LARYNX: (2) nit-ac., phos.; *cough, during:* (2) phos.; *swallowing, when:* (1) Mang.; (2) brom.; *extending to ear when swallowing:* (1) Mang. TRACHEA: (1) Stann. TEARING, LARYNX, *coughing, on:* (2) all-c.

Paralysis, LARYNX: (1) Caust.; (2) alum., gels., lach., plb.

Phthisis, LARYNX: Spong., Stann.; (2) arg-m., caust., dros., hep., iod., kali-bi., kali-i., phos.; *short hacking cough and loss of voice:* (1) Stann.; *singers and public speakers:* (2) arg-m. TRACHEA: (2) ars., dros., stann.

Plug, LARYNX: (1) Spong. TRACHEA: (2) lach.

Polypi, LARYNX: (2) sang.

Pulsating, LARYNX: (2) all-c.

Rattling, LARYNX: (1) Brom.; (2) ant-t. TRACHEA: (1) Ant-t., Hep., Ip.

Roughness: (1) Carb-v.; (2) caust., mang., phos., seneg., stann., sul. LARYNX: (1) Mang., Spong., Rhus-t.; (2) hep., phos.; *morning:* (2) calc.

Scraping, LARYNX: (1) Cham., Puls., Rhus-t.; (2) caust., hep., spong.; *evening:* (2) carb-v., coc-c.; *coughing, from:* (1) Brom.; (2) coc-c.

Sensitive LARYNX: (2) acon., caust., lach., phos.; *cold air, to:* (1) Hep.; *pressure, to:* (1) Phos.; *sound of the piano, to:* (1) Calc.; *touch, to:* (1) Lach., Spong., Phos., Acon.; (2) hep. TRACHEA, *cold air, to:* (2) rumex; *touch, to:* (2) hep.

Sulphur *vapor, as from:* (1) Ars.; (2) puls.

Supports LARYNX *on coughing:* (2) acon., dros.

Swollen LARYNX: (1) Bell., (2) hep., lach.

Tickling, LARYNX: (2) all-c., cham., nux-v., phos., puls., stict.; *talking, while:* (2) phos. TRACHEA: (2) nux-v., phos., puls., spong., stann.

Ulceration, LARYNX: (2) calc., cinnb., syphil.

Velvety *sensation:* (1) Phos.; (2) hep.

Voice, *bass:* (1) Dros.; *changeable:* (1) Arum-t.; *cracked:* (2) spong.; *evening:* (2) spong.; *singing, when:* (2) graph.; *croaking:* (1) Stram.; *deep:* (1) Dros., Carb-v.; (2) stann., verb.; *hoarseness:* (1) Caust., Carb-v., Dros., Spong., Phos., Calc.; (2) arg-n., arum-t., bell., kali-bi.; *morning:* (1) Caust., Calc., Phos.; *evening:* (1) Carb-v., Phos.; (2) sul.; *coryza, during:* (1) Merc., Caust., Carb-v., Mang., Phos.; *croup, after:* (2) carb-v.; *crying, when:* (1) Bell.; *damp weather, in:* (2) carb-v.; *measles, after:* (2) carb-v., dros.; *mucus in larynx:* (1) Samb.; *overuse of the voice:* (1) Arum-t., Rhus-t., Caps.; (2) arn., caust., phos.; *painful:* (2) phos., stict.; *painless:* (1) Calc., Carb-v.; (2) caust., dig.; *singing, while:* (1) Arum-t., Agar.; *speech, preventing:* (1) Phos.; *sudden:* (2) bell., spong.; *talking:* (1) Arum-t., Arg-m., Rhus-t.; (2) phos.; *walking in open air, after, against the wind:* (2) nicc., nux-m.; *hollow:* (1) Dros., Spong., Verat.; (2) arum-t.; *husky:* (1) Dros., Phos.; (2) spong., sul.; *indistinct:* (1) Brom.; *inflexible:* (1) Stram.; *lost:* (1) Caust., Phos., Brom., Arg-m., Arg-n., Carb-v.; (2) alum., ant-c., kali-bi., lach., puls., spong., stram.; *morning:* (2) brom.; *waking, on:* (2) ail.; *evening:* (2) carb-v., phos.; *night:* (2) carb-v.; *air, damp, cold:* (2)

rumex; *cold, exposure to:* (2) caust., rumex; *fright, from:* (2) acon., gels., op.; *hysterical:* (2) ign., nux-m.; *menses, during:* (2) gels.; *mucus in larynx, from:* (2) bar-c.; *overheated, from being:* (2) ant-c.; *overuse of:* (2) caust.; *painless:* (2) phos.; *paralysis, from:* (1) Caust.; (2) gels., lach., plb.; *prolonged talking, from:* (2) phos.; *singers:* (1) Arg-m.; *sudden:* (1) Caust.; *nasal:* (1) Kali-bi.; (2) phos.; *rough:* (1) Bell., Carb-v., Phos., Kali-bi.; (2) brom., caust., hyos., puls., spong., sul.; *morning:* (2) calc.; *air, open, in:* (1) Mang.; *shrieking:* (1) Arum-t.; *squeaking:* (1) Stram.; *toneless:* (1) Dros., Stram.; *tremulous:* (2) ign., nux-m., phos.; *weak:* (1) Stann., Hep., Verat.; (2) carb-v., chin., ign., phos-ac., phos., spong.; *whining:* (2) cina.

COUGH.

Cough *in general:* (1) Bry., Phos., Rumex, Dros., Sul., Puls., Calc.; (2) acon., ars., bell., coc-c., hyos., sang., sep., stann.

Daytime: (1) Phos., Euphr., Nat-s.; (2) am-c., lach., *expectoration, copious, greenish, salty, agg. morning:* (2) stann.; *night, and:* (2) bell., ign., phos.; spong.; *only:* (1) Euphr.; (2) phos.

Morning: (1) Nux-v., Ars., Puls.; (2) calc., chin., lyc., phos.; *bed, in:* (2) caust., phos.; *night, and:* (2) caust.; *rising, on:* (2) ars., cina, ferr., phos.; *waking, on:* (1) Rumex; (2) sil.

Noon, *lying down, amel.:* (1) Mang.

Afternoon: (2) bell., chel., sang.; *4 to 8 p. m.:* (1) Lyc.; 4 *until bed time:* (2) mang.

Evening: (1) Puls., Ars.; (2) bell., caps., lyc., merc.; *bed, in, agg.:* (1) Ars., Merc., Ign.; (2) lyc., puls., sep., sul.; *lying down, on:* (1) Puls., Sep., Hyos.; (2) bell.; *must sit up:* (1) Puls.; *midnight, until:* (2) puls., rhus-t.; *sleep, after going to:* (2) lach.; *on going to:* (2) hep.

Night: (1) Acon., Ars., Bell., Cham., Puls.; (2) graph., kali-c., lach., merc., sep., sil., sul.; *waking from the cough:* (1) Hyos., Sep.; *3 a. m.:* (1) Kali-c.; *3 to 4 a. m.:* (2) am-c., kali-c.

Air, *cold, agg.:* (2) all-c., ars., caust., phos., rumex; *walking in, agg.:* (2) ars., phos., rumex; *damp cold agg.:* (2) lach.; *open, agg.:* (1) Ars.; (2) lach., phos., sul.; *amel.:* (1) Bry., Coc-c.; (2) iod., mag-p.; *warm, amel.:* (2) rumex, seneg.

Anger, *from:* (2) ant-t., cham., staph.

Asthmatic: (1) Ip., Ars., Ant-t., Cupr.; (2) cina, dros., hep., nux-v.

Barking: (1) Acon., Bell., Hep., Spong.; (2) dros., rumex; *day and night:* (2) spong.; *drinking cold water, amel.:* (2) coc-c., caust.; *loud:* (2) acon.

Bed, *warm, on becoming, in, agg. or excites:* (1) Puls., Caust.

Breathing *deep agg.:* (2) hep., lyc., rumex, squil.

Chill, *before:* (1) Rhus-t.; *during:* (2) ars., phos., rhus-t., sabad.

Choking (*compare* "*Suffocative*"): (2) hep., kali-c., lach.; *morning, rising, after:* (1) Cina; *sleep, as soon as one falls into a sound:* (1) Lach.; *after first sleep:* (2) aral.

Cold, *on becoming, arm or hand, agg.:* (1) Hep., Rhus-t.; *single part;* (1) Hep., Rhus-t.; *drinks amel.:* (1) Caust., Cupr.; (2) coc-c., op.; *walking in, agg.:* (2) phos.

Concussive (*see* "*Shaking*"): (1) Ign., Merc.; (2) carb-v., puls.

Consciousness, *loss of, with:* (3) cupr.

Constant: (2) spong.; *evening:* (1) Puls.; *lying down after:* (1) Puls.; *night:* (1) Sep.; *lying down agg.:* (1) Sep.; *waking:* (1) Sep.; *lying agg., sitting up amel.:* (1) Hyos., Puls.

Constriction, *larynx, agg.:* (2) ip.

Continued *coughing, agg.:* (1) Ign.

Convulsive: (1) Ambr., Sep.; (2) bell., hyos., rumex; *evening:* (2) carb-v.

Coryza, *with:* (2) euphr., sul.

Coughing *agg.:* (1) Ign.
Crawling, *sensation of, larynx:* (1) Con.; (2) dros.; *throat-pit, from:* (1) Sang.
Croupy: (1) Acon., Spong., Hep., Iod., Phos., Lach., Samb.
Crowing: (1) Samb.; (2) spong.
Crumb, *feeling as of a, in larynx, from:* (2) lach.
Crying *agg.:* (2) arn.; *before:* (2) arn.; *during:* (1) Hep.; (2) bell., cina.
Debauch, *after:* (2) nux-v.
Deep: (1) Stann.; (2) hep., verb.; *noon, toward amel.:* (1) Mang.; *evening.:* (1) Verat.; *lying down amel.:* (1) Mang.
Deep *enough, sensation as though he could not cough, to start mucus:* (1) Caust.
Dentition, *during:* (2) cham.
Distressing, *morning and evening, on going to sleep:* (2) brom., lach.
Drinking, *after:* (2) ars., phos.; *amel.:* (2) coc-c., spong.
Dry: (1) Bry., Phos., Acon., Ars., Rumex, Nux-v., Spong.; (2) alum., hyos., ign., lach., petr.; *day-time, night, and:* (2) spong.: *morning, menses, before:* (1) Zinc.; *evening:* (2) brom., ign., phos.; *loose in morning:* (1) Squil.; *lying down, agg.:* (1) Puls., Sang., Bell., Hyos.; *sleep, on going to:* (2) hep.; *night:* (1) Phos., Spong., Sul.; (2) bell., merc.; *sitting up amel.:* (1) Hyos., Puls.; *waking, on:* (1) Sul.; (2) puls.; *midnight, daybreak, until:* (1) Nux-v.; *lying on back agg.:* (2) nux-v.; *on side amel.:* (2) nux-v.; *3 a. m.:* (2) am-c., kali-c.;

drinking amel.: (1) Spong.; (2) coc-c.; *eating amel.:* (2) spong.; *fever during:* (1) Acon., Sabad.; (2) bry., ip., kali-c., nat-m., nux-v., phos.; *flatus, discharge up and down, amel.; must sit up also:* (1) Sang.; *lying, while:* (1) Hyos., Puls.; *back, on, agg.:* (2) phos.; *midnight:* (2) nux-v.; *amel.:* (2) mang.; *side, left, agg.:* (1) Phos.; *measles, after:* (2) dros., stict.; *menses, before:* (1) Zinc.; (2) sul.; *morning:* (1) Zinc.; *during:* (1) Zinc.; (2) bry., graph.; *suppressed, from:* (2) cop.; *morning:* (2) cop.; *reading aloud:* (1) Phos.; (2) mang.; *scraping in larynx, from:* (2) bell., brom., coc-c., puls.; *sitting amel.:* (2) sang.; *sitting up at night amel.:* (2) puls.; *sleep, during:* (1) Cham., Lach.; (2) rhus-t; *tickling in larynx, from:* (2) bell., brom., lach., puls.; *waking, on:* (1) Sul.; (2) puls., sang.; *warm room, on entering a:* (1) Bry.; (2) nat-c.

Dryness, *fauces agg.:* (1) Dros.; (2) phyt.; *spots in causes:* (1) Con.

Dry *spot, larynx in, from:* (1) Con.; *throat in, from:* (2) cimic.

Dust, *as from:* (1) Puls., Lyc.; (2) am-c., ign., sul.; *in throat-pit:* (2) ign.

Dyspnœa: (1) Ip., Ars., Ant-t., Cupr., Nux-v., Dros.; (2) hep., op.

Eating *agg.:* (1) Kali-bi.; (2) rumex; *after:* (1) Nux-v., Bry.; (2) ant-t., ars., ferr., sep.; *until he vomits:* (2) mez.

Exertion *agg.:* (2) bry., nux-v.; *violent, agg.:* (1) Puls.; *mental:* (2) nux-v.

Exhausting: (1) Ars., Stann.; (2) carb-v., cupr., kali-c., phos.; *evening*: (2) kali-c., sil.; *night*: (1) Puls.; (2) caust.; *bed, in*: (2) caust.; *sleep, disturbing*: (1) Puls.

Expiration *agg.*: (2) acon., carb-v., caust.

Eyes, *closing, from*: (2) hep.

Fears *to, and seems to avoid it as long as possible, children with bronchial catarrh*: (2) phos.

Fever, *during*: (2) acon., ars., calc., con., ip., kali-c., nat-m., nux-v., phos., sabad.

Fire, *looking into, agg.*: (2) ant-c.

Flesh, *sensation as if cough would tear a piece of, from the throat*: (2) phos.

Forcible *expectoration tenacious mucus amel.*: (2) phos.

Gonorrhœa, *suppressed, after*: (2) med., thuj.

Grasping *throat during*: (2) acon., all-c.; *larynx involuntarily at every cough, feels as though larynx would be torn*: (2) all-c.

Hacking: (1) Phos., Nat-m., Ars.; (2) alum., sang.; *afternoon*: (1) Sang.; *evening*: (1) Ign., Sang.; (2) sul.; *bed, in*: (1) Sep.; (2) rhus-t., sul.; *lying down, after*: (1) Ign., Sang., Sep.; *dinner, after*: (1) Hep.; *dryness in throat, from*: (1) Sang.; *eating, while*: (2) hep.; *lying down, while*: (2) ign.

Hands, *must hold chest with both, while*: (1) Arn., Bry.; (2) dros., eup-per., nat-p.; *holding pit of stomach amel.*: (2) croc.

Heated, *on becoming, agg.*: (1) Puls.; (2) bry.

Hectic: (2) phos., stann.

Hoarse: (1) Bell., Hep., All-c., Stann.; (2) calc., carb-v., caust., rhus-t.; *croupy:* (2) brom.

Hollow: (1) Bell., Verat.; (2) caust., phos., verb.; *morning:* (2) caust., ign.; *bed, in:* (2) phos.; *waking, on:* (1) Ign.; *night:* (2) phos.

Hysterical *attack of, in women:* (2) ign.

Icy *cold air, in air passages, sensation of, from:* (2) cor-r.

Inability *to:* (2) dros.; *amel. by pressure of hand on pit of stomach:* (2) dros.

Irritation *in air passages from:* (2) caust., cham.; *increases the more one coughs:* (1) Ign.; *in throat-pit from:* (1) Ign.

Laughing *agg.:* (2) arg-m., phos., stann.

Lying *agg.:* (1) Hyos., Puls.; sang.; (2) apis, ars., bry., sul.; *morning on rising:* (1) Euphr.; *noon, amel.:* (1) Mang.; *evening:* (1) Puls.; (2) bell., kali-c., sep.; *must sit up:* (2) puls.; *midnight wakens him:* (1) Apis; *before:* (2) aral.; *amel.:* (1) Mang.; (2) thuj.; *back, on, agg.:* (2) nat-m., nux-v., phos.; *amel.:* (2) mang.; *better than either side, though worse lying on left side:* (2) phos.; *bed, agg.:* (1) Phos., Sul.; (2) hyos., puls., rhus-t.; *head low, with, agg.:* (1) Chin.; *raised, amel.:* (1) Chin.; *only when first lying down; was obliged to sit up and cough it out, when had rest:* (1) Con.; *rising up amel.:* (2) puls., rhus-t., sabad.; *side, right, agg.:* (1) Merc., Stann.; (2) cina; *left, agg.:* (2) phos., thuj.; *turning to right side amel.:* (2) thuj.

Measles, *after:* (1) Dros.; (2) stict.

Meditation, *from:* (2) nux-v.

Menses, *before, morning:* (1) Zinc.; *evening:* (2) sul.; *bed, in, sitting up amel.:* (2) sul.; *beginning of, at:* (2) phos.; *during:* (2) sep., zinc.; *evening, every:* (2) sul.

Motion *agg.:* (2) ars., bry., nux-v., phos., sil., stann.; *amel.* (*compare* "*Rest*"): (2) rhus-t.; *chest, of, agg.:* (1) Chin., Nux-v., Stann.

Mucus *in trachea, sensation of, from:* (1) Stann.

Overpowering, *as if larynx were tickled by a feather in evening before sleep:* (1) Lyc.

Painful: (1) Bry.; (2) nat-s.; *night:* (2) rhus-t.; *midnight, waking before:* (2) rhus-t.

Paroxysmal: (1) Bell, Dros., Cina; (2) carb-v., hep; hyos., rumex, stann., verat.; *waking, after:* (1, Rumex, con.; *afternoon:* (2) chel.; *4 p. m.:* (2) chel) *night:* (1) Rumex; *midnight, before:* (1) Rumex; *11 p. m.:* (1) Rumex; *lying down, after:* (1) Rumex; *sleep, after:* (2) lach.; *after:* (2) dros.; *attacks follow one another quickly:* (1) Dros.; *consisting of long coughs:* (1) Cupr.; *gagging, with:* (1) Dros.; *perspiration, and with:* (1) Ars.; *stomach, laying hand on pit of, amel.:* (2) croc.; *suffocation, suddenly on swallowing:* (1) Brom.

Persistent: (2) cupr., hyos., nux-v.; *midnight, lying on back, agg.; lying on side, amel.:* (2) nux-v.

Plug, *sensation of a, moving up and down in throat, from:* (2) calc.

Pressure *upon larynx, from:* (1) Lach.; *of fingers on trachea, from:* (2) lach.

Racking: (1) Caust., Merc., Nux-v., Sul., Puls.; (2) carb-v., hyos.

Rattling: (1) Ip.; (2) ant-t., coc-c., kali-s., op., puls., sep., stann., sul.; *eating, while:* (2) phos.

Reading *aloud agg.:* (1) Phos.; (2) spong., stann.

Rigidity *of body, with:* (1) Ip., Cupr.

Rising, *before:* (1) Nux-v.

Scraped *feeling and roughness in larynx, from:* (1) Nux-v.

Scraping, *fauces, agg.:* (1) Dros.; *larynx, in, from:* (1) Brom., Puls.; (2) bell., coc-c.; *throat, in, from:* (2) alumn., bell.

Short: (1) Coff., Acon.; (2) bell., bry., caust., ign., lach., nux-v., phos.; *evening:* (1) Ign.; *interruption of respiration in upper trachea:* (1) Ign.

Sibilant: (2) spong.; *and dry, like a saw driven through a pine board:* (2) spong.

Singing *agg.:* (2) phos., spong.

Sit up, *must:* (1) Phos., Puls.; *as soon as cough commences:* (2) bry.; *and cough it out, when had rest:* (1) Con.

Sitting *up amel. (see "Lying"):* (1) Hyos., Puls.; (2) sang.

Sleep, *before:* (1) Sul.; *during:* (1) Lach.; (2) acon., cham., rhus-t.; *after:* (2) lach.; *going to, on:* (2) hep.; *preventing:* (1) Puls.; (2) lyc., sep.; *waking from:* (1) Phos.; (2) hyos., lach., sang.

Smoking *agg.:* (2) ign.

Sneezing, *with:* (2) bell.

Spasmodic (*compare "Convulsive," "Paroxysmal"*):- (1) Cupr., Dros., Hyos., Ip., Nux-v.; (2) bry., carb-v., puls.

Springs *up, child, and clings to those around; calls*

for help in a hoarse voice, or bends backward and grasps at larynx: (2) ant-t.

Stomach, *seems to come from the:* (1) Sep.; *turned inside out, feeling as if:* (2) puls.

Sudden: (1) Squil.; *morning:* (1) Squil.; *evening;* (2) am-br.

Suffocative: (1) Ip., Dros.; (2) ant-t., chin., cina, nux-v., samb., sul.; *evening, child becomes quite stiff and blue in the face:* (1) Ip.; *midnight, after:* (2) kali-c.; *5 a. m.:* (2) kali-c.

Sulphur *fumes or vapor, sensation of agg.:* (1) Ars., Ign., Puls.

Sun *agg.:* (2) ant-c.

Talking *agg.:* (2) chin., hep., lach., phos., spong.; *inability to speak, with:* (2) cimic., cupr.

Tickling: (1) Cham., Nat-m., Nux-v., Acon.; (2) ip., lach., phos., sep., staph.; *air passages, in, from:* (1) Cham., Acon., Nux-v., Nat-m.; (2) iod., ip., rumex, sep., spong., staph.; *spot, small:* (2) con.; *throat, in, from:* (1) Phos., Cham., Nat-m., Rumex; (2) acon.; *throat-pit, in, from:* (2) cham., rumex, sang., sil.; *tonsils, below:* (2) am-br.; *trachea, in, from:* (2) acon., kali-bi.

Tormenting: (2) caust., nux-v., phos., squil.

Touching *throat agg.:* (1) Lach.; (2) bell., rumex.

Uncovering *agg.:* (1) Hep.; *feet or head agg.:* (1) Sil.; *hands agg.:* (1) Hep.; (2) rhus-t.

Vaccination, *after:* (2) thuj.

Vexation, *after:* (1) Ign., Staph., Cham.; (2) nat-m.

Violent, *morning:* (1) Squil.; *night, 3 a. m.:* (1) Kali-c.; *perspiration, causing profuse:* (1) Merc.; (2) ant-t., ars., carb-v., chin., hep., phos.

Warm, *fluids agg.:* (2) coc-c.; *food agg.:* (2) coc-c., kali-c., puls.; *amel.:* (2) spong.; *room agg.:* (1) Coc-c.; (2) bry., dros., nat-c.; *entering, from open air, agg.:* (2) bry., coc-c., nat-c.; *going from, to cold air, or vice versa, agg.:* (1) Phos.; (2) rumex; *to open air, agg.:* (1) Phos.; (2) acon.

Wheezing : (2) ant-t., ip., kali-bi., samb., spong.

Whistling : (2) sang.

Whooping : (2) ant-t., arn., bell., cina, coc-c., cupr., dros., meph., nux-v., sul., verat.

Winter : (2) cham., psor.

EXPECTORATION.

Morning: (1) Bry., Phos., Calc., Puls., Sep., Hep., Squil.; (2) lyc., sul. ac.; *bed, in:* (2) calc.; *waking, after:* (2) sul.

Night: (1) Sep.

Acid: (1) Nux-v., Calc., Phos.; (2) kali-c.

Acrid: (2) puls., sil.

Albuminous: (2) ars., seneg., stann.

Balls, *in shape of:* (1) Stann.; (2) arg-n., Coc-c.

Batter, *breaks and flies like thin:* (2) phos.

Bed, *in:* (2) phos.; *sitting up in, on:* (2) phos.

Blackish: (2) chin., elaps, nux-v.

Bloody, *spitting of blood:* (1) Acon., Ferr., Ip., Arn., Phos., Puls., Sul.; (2) bry., calc., carb-v., ham., mill.; *morning, menses, during:* (1) Zinc.; *acrid:* (1) Kali-c., Sil.; *black:* (1) Elaps; *bright-red color:* (1) Bell., Hyos.; (2) dulc., sabin.; *brown:* (1) Bry., Carb-v.; (2) calc., rhus-t.; *dark:* (1) Cham., Croc., Nux-v.; *fall, after a:* (2) ferr-ph., mill.; *menses, before:* (2) zinc.; *during*: (2) phos.; *in points and copious:* (1) Laur.; *streaked:* (1) Bry., Ferr.; (2) arn., chin., ip., phos.; *viscid:* (1) Croc.

Bluish: (2) kali-bi.

Brick-dust, *color* (*See "Rusty"*): (1) Phos.

Brownish: (2) carb-v.

Burned, *when dry on the floor,* looks as *if:* (2) phos.

Casts, *fibro-elastic:* (2) kali-bi.

Cool (*cold*): (2) cor-r., phos.

Copious: (1) Stann., Puls., Lyc., Calc., Sep.; (2) ars., carb-v., chin., euph., kali-c., phos., sil., sul.

Difficult: (2) chel., coc-c., lach., phos.

Easy: (1) Stann.

Flies *forcibly out of mouth*: (2) bad , chel., kali-c.

Frequent: (2) puls., sep., stann.

Frothy: (1) Ars.; (2) kali-i.

Grayish: (1) Lyc.; (2) ambr., calc.

Greenish: (1) Kali-i., Puls.; (2) lyc., sep., stann.; *morning*: (2) lyc.; *lying down, while*: (2) psor.

Mucous: (2) ars., calc., chin., lyc., par., phos., stann.; *tough*: (2) ars., kali-bi., seneg.

Odor *of an old catarrh*: (2) puls., sul.; *fetid*: (2) calc., sang., sep., stann.; *offensive*: (1) Sang.; (2) calc., sep., stann.

Purulent: (1) Sil., Calc., Chin., Kali-c., Lyc., Phos., Sep.

Rusty: (1) Bry.; (2) phos., rhus-t., sang.

Scanty: (2) phos., stann.

Stringy: (1) Kali-bi.; (2) coc-c., hydr.

Swallow, *must, what has been loosened*: (2) caust., kali-i., spong.

Taste *bitter*: (1) Puls., Cham.; (2) sep.; *greasy*: (1) Caust., Puls.; (2) sil.; *nauseous*: (1) Puls.; (2) ip., stann.; *putrid*: (2) carb-v., puls., stann.; *salty*: (1) Sep., Kali-iod.; (2) ars., lyc.; *sweetish*: (1) Stann., Phos.

Tenacious: (2) carb-v., coc-c., kali-bi.

Thick: (2) stann.

Whitish: (1) Lyc., Sep.; (2) phos., sul.

Yellow: (1) Puls., Calc., Lyc., Phos., Stann., Sil.; *morning*: (2) calc., calc-ph., ph-ac.

RESPIRATION.

Abdominal : (1) Ant-t.

Accelerated : (1) Acon., Bell., Bry., Ars., Phos., Sub., Ant-t.; (2) carb-v., chel., gels., ip., lyc., sep.; *cough, during paroxysm of:* (1) Dros.; *exercise, during:* (2) calc.

Anxious : (1) Acon., Ars., Phos.; (2) bar-m., chel., ip., nat-m., puls., spong.

Arrested : (1) Bry., Cupr., Samb.; *night:* (1) Lyc.; *air, in fresh:* (1) Psor.; *coughing:* (1) Ip.; Cupr., Cina, Ars., Ant-t., Dros., Nux-v.; (2) alumn., cor-r., samb.; *sleep, on going to:* (1) Lach., Grind., Op., Dig.; *sleep during:* (1) Lach., Op.; *stitches in rectum:* (1) Sul.; *umbilicus, pain in,* from*:* (2) nux-v.; *walking, when:* (2) calc.; *against the wind:* (2) calc.

Asphyxia : (1) Ant-t.; *new-born infant:* (1) Ant-t., Camph.; (2) bell., laur.

Asthmatic : (1) Ip., Ars., Lobel., Samb.; (2) ambr., kali-c., meph., nat-s., puls., seneg., sep., stram., sul.; *morning:* (1) kali-c.; *evening:* (1) Puls.; (2) phos.; *night:* (1) Ars., Puls.; (2) ant-t., carb-v., chel., sul.; *midnight, after:* (1) Ars., Samb.; *must spring out of bed:* (1) Ars., Samb.; 2 *a. m.:* (1) Ars.; (2) rumex; *3 a. m.:* (1) Kali-c.; (2) cupr.; *4 to 5 a. m.:* (2) nat-s.; *air, draught of, agg.:* (2) sil.; *anger, after a fit of:* (1) Cham.; *bending head backwards amel:* (1) Spong.; *children:* (1) Ip., Cham., Samb.; (2) puls.; *cold, from taking:* (1) Spong.; *cold air agg.:* (2) nux-v.;

amel.: (1) Puls.; *water agg.:* (2) meph.; *emotions, after:* (2) acon.; coff., gels., ign.; *eruptions, after suppressed:* (1) Ars., Puls.; *flatulence, from:* (2) carb-v., cham., chin., lyc., sul.; *hay asthma:* (2) ars., carb-v., iod., kali-i., naja, nat-s., sin-n.; *hysterical:* (1) Mosch., Nux-m., Puls., *menses, after suppression of:* (2) puls.; *moon, full, agg.:* (1) Spong.; (2) calc.; *old people, in:* (1) Ars.; (2) ambr., carb-v.; *rose cold, following:* (2) sang.; *sailors as soon as they go ashore:* (1) Brom.; *spasmodic:* (1) Ip., Lobel.; (2) aral., bell., cupr., kali-c., lach., spong., valer.; *wet weather, in:* (2) dulc., nat-s.

Cold *(breath):* (1) Camph., Carb-v., Verat.; *during chill:* (1) Carb-v.

Deep: (1) Bry., Ign., Op., Phos., Ip.; (2) caps., dig., selen., sil.; *ameliorates:* (2) cupr., ign., seneg., spig., stann.; *desire to breathe:* (1) Bry., Ign., Nat-s., Cact.; (2) phos., seneg.; *impossible:* (1) Ars.; *need frequent:* (1) Ign., Lach., Sul.; (2) calc.; *running, after:* (2) hep.

Difficult: (1) Ars., Ip., Phos., Nat-s., Lach., Puls., Sul.; (2) apis, cact., chlor., crot-t., cupr-ac., kali-c., lobel., lyc., naja, nux-m., op., spong., squil., stann.; *morning:* (2) lach., nux-v., phos.; *evening:* (2) ars., carb-v., phos., psor., puls., sul.; *anxiety, with:* (2) phos.; *in bed:* (2) ars., carb-v., phos., sep.; *night, during:* (1) Ars., Phos.; (2) puls., sul.; *in bed:* (1) Ars.; *lying on back:* (2) sul.; *midnight:* (2) ars.; *after:* (1) Ars., Samb.; (2) dros., spong.; *1 to 4 a. m.:* (2) syph.; *2 a. m.:* (1) Ars.; *3 a. m.:* (1) Samb.; *frequent attacks* *until 4 a. m.:* (1) Samb.; *air, when in cold, amel.:* (2) bry., puls.; *in open air, agg.:* (1) Psor.; *amel.:* (1) Puls., Apis, Nat-m., Sul.; *fanned, wants to be:* (1) Carb-v.; (2) ferr.; *anger, from a fit of:* (1) Cham.; *arms close to body agg.:* (2) psor.; *lies with arms outstretched:* (2) psor.; *on bending backward:* (1) Sul.; *ascending:* (1) Ars., Calc., Nat-m.; *bending arm backwards, on:* (1) Sul.; *chest, from pain in, from rheumatism:* (2) abrot., kalm.; *children:* (2) ambr.; *chill, during:* (1) Apis; (2) nat-m.; *coition, during:* (2) ambr., staph.; *toward end of:* (2) staph.; *cough, during:* (2) alumn., ars.; *dust, as from:* (1) Ars., Sil.; (2) calc., hep.; *eating, after:* (1) Lach., Phos., Puls.; (2) sul.; *warm food:* (2) lobel.; *eating amel.:* (2) spong.; *emissions, after:* (1) Staph.; (2) phos.; *excitement agg.:* (2) puls.; *exercising, while:* (1) Ip., Ars.; (2) phos., sil., stann.; *exertion, after:* (1) Ars., Spong., Lobel.; (2) carb-v., ip., phos., stann., sul.; *with hands and arms:* (1) Lach.; *mental:* (2) nat-m.; *expectoration amel.:* (1) Ant-t.; (2) grind., zinc.; *expiration:* (2) chlor., ip., samb.; *almost impossible:* (2) chlor.; *fainting, with:* (1) Carb-v.; (2) chin., spong.; *fanned, wants to be:* (1) Carb-v.; *flatulence, from:* (2) carb-v., zinc.; *fright, after:* (2) samb.; *heart, during pain in:* (2) cact., psor., spong.; *complaints and urinary troubles:* (1) Laur.; *heat, with:* (1) Apis; (2) kali-c.; *hysterical:* (2) ign., mosch.; *inspiration:* (1) Samb.; (2) calc., phos.; *rapid expiration:* (2) kali-c., sang.; *larynx, touching, spasms of:* (1) Chlor., Gels., Ign.; (2) laur., mosch., samb.; *lung paralysis:* (1) Ant-t., Chin.; (2) laur., phos.; *in old people:* (2) bar-c., carb-v., chin.; *lying, while:* (1) Ars.; (2) ant-t., hep., lach., merc., phos., puls., sul.; *amel.:* (2) dig., laur., nux-v., psor.; *head low, with the:* (2) chin., spong., spig.; *on the back:* (1) Lyc.; (2) phos., puls.; *amel.:* (1) Cact.; (2) kalm.; *with shoulders elevated amel.:* (2) spig.; *impossible:* (1) Ars., Apis; (2) ant-t., lach., nux-v., puls., sul.; *menses, before:* (1) Zinc.; (2) sul.; *during:* (1) Spong.; (2) lach.; *after:* (2) nat-m.; *suppressed, with:* (1) Puls.; *motion:* (2) bry., nat-s., spong.; *of arms agg.:* (1) Lach.; *open, wants doors and windows:* (1) Puls., Sul., Apis, Lach.; *must sit by the window:* (2) chel.; *palpitation, during:* (2) cact., calc., kali-c., psor., spig., spong.; *periodical attacks:* (1) Cact.; *raising arms:* (1) Spig.; *rest, during:* (1) Ferr.; *riding on horseback agg.:* (2) meph.; *sitting:* (2) lach., phos., psor.; *bent forward amel.:* (1) Lach., Spong.; (2) kali-c.; *with head bent forward on knees amel.:* (1) Kali-c.; *sleep, during:* (1) Lach., Grind.; (2) carb-v., kali-c., op., sul.; *awakened to avoid suffocation, must be:* (1) Op.; *after agg.:* (1) Lach.; (2) sep., phos.; *falling asleep, when:* (1) Grind., Lach., Op., Dig.; (2) spong.; *waking one from:* (1) Grind., Lach., Op.; *night:* (2) samb.; *smoke, as from:* (2) brom.; *stomach, pain in, from:* (1) Ars.; *talking:* (1) Lach., Spong.; (2) caust.; *amel.:* (2) ferr.; *throat, constriction about:* (1)

Lach., Apis; *touching the:* (1) Lach.; (2) apis; *turning in bed:* (1) Ars.; (2) sul.; *umbilicus, pain in:* (2) nux-v.; *uterus, pressure in:* (1) Sep.; *walking:* (1) Calc.; (2) ars., carb-v., dig., kali-c., nat-s.; *in the open air:* (2) ars., sul.; *amel.:* (2) dros.; *rapidly:* (1) Phos., Puls.; (2) cupr., kali-c.; *amel.:* (2) sep.; *against the wind:* (2) calc., nux-m.; *warm room, in a:* (1) Apis, Puls.; (2) sul.; *becomes deathly pale and must remain quiet:* (2) am-c.; *water, when standing in:* (2) nux-m.; *weakness of respiratory organs:* (1) Stann.; *working:* (2) nux-m.

Gasping: (1) Apis, Lyc.; (2) ant-t., ars., dig., med., mosch., naja, phos., spong.; *cough, before:* (2) brom.; *during:* (2) ant-t.; *inspiration, expiration long and slow:* (2) ant-t.; *whooping cough:* (2) cor-r.

Hot *breath:* (1) Acon.; (2) bell., cham., phos.

Impeded, *chest, by constriction in:* (1) Cact.; (2) caps.; *stitches in:* (2) bry.; *thrusts in left, toward heart:* (2) sul.; *coffee, after:* (2) cham.; *cough, during:* (2) cupr., ip.; *covering nose or mouth:* (2) arg-n., lach.; *gagging in esophagus:* (2) cimx.; *heart, stitches in:* (2) cact., naja; *stopped, as if:* (1) Dig.; *pains take away the breath:* (1) Bry.; *stomach, pressure:* (2) nux-m.; *constriction:* (2) cact.; *pain in:* (2) ars.; *stooping, from:* (2) calc.; *talking, while:* (2) caust.; *walking:* (1) Phos.

Intermittent: (1) Ant-t.; *sleep, during:* (2) ant-t.

Irregular: (1) Dig., Cupr., Op., Morph.; (2) ail., ang., bell.; *at one time slow, at another time hurried:* (2) ign.; *sleep, during:* (2) ign.

Jerking, *inspiration:* (1) Ox-ac.

Long: (2) op.; *expiration:* (2) chlor., op.; *slow, wheezing expiration:* (2) sep.

Loud: (2) calc., cham., chin., kali-bi., lach., phos., samb., spong., sul.; *sleep, in:* (1) Puls.

Moaning: (2) ant-t., phos.

Mouth open: (1) Bell.; (2) lyc., phos.

Painful: (1) Ran-b.

Panting: (1) Phos., Verat-v.; (2) ant-t., bry., cina, lyc., spong.; *ascending, stairs:* (1) Calc.

Rattling: (1) Ant-t., Lyc., Kali-s., Puls., Phos., Chin.; (2) ars., calc., carb-v., cupr., dulc., hep., ip., stann., sul.; *sleep, during:* (2) hep.

Rough: (1) Bry.; (2) hep.; *crowing:* (1) Bry., Samb.; (2) cupr., gels.; *sawing:* (2) spong.

Short: (1) Ant-t., Ars., Carb-v., Phos., Bry., Sul.; (2) bell., caust., chel., sil., stann.; *evening:* (1) Sul.; *6 p. m.:* (1) Rhus-t.; *ascending height agg.:* (1) Calc.; *bending arms backward:* (1) Sul.; *cough, during:* (1) Stann.; *eating, after:* (1) Anac.; *exertion, on:* (1) Ars., Lyc., Nat-m.; *expectoration, from suppressed:* (1) Ant-t.; *fever, during:* (1) Apis; *heat, from:* (2) apis; *lying, while:* (2) ars.; *amel.:* (2) psor.; *moon, increase of, agg.:* (2) phell.; *motion:* (1) Bry.; (2) lyc.; *of hands, after, agg.:* (2) lach.; *riding, amel. by:* (2) psor.; *sleep, during:* (2) acon., hep., lyc.; *after weeping:* (2) calc.; *suppressed eruptions, after:* (1) Apis; *talking much, after:* (1) Sul., Spig.; *walking, while:*

(1) Calc., Sul.; (2) ars.; *rapidly:* (1) Nat-m.; (2) sul.; *in open air:* (1) Sul.

Sighing: (1) Ign., Bry., Dig., Op., Secale; (2) calc-p., ip., stram.; *sleep, during:* (2) sul.

Slow: (1) Bell., Op.; (2) dig., gels., lach.; *morning:* (2) lach.; *night:* (2) lach.

Snoring: (1) Op.; *chill, during:* (1) Op.; *expiration during:* (2) op.; *heat, during:* (1) Op.

Sobbing: (2) ign.; *in sleep:* (1) Aur.

Stertorous: (1) Op., Am-c.; (2) ant-t., nux-m.; *puffing expiration, with:* (2) lach.; *sleep, during:* (1) Op., Puls.; *stupefaction and crying out as with a sharp pain:* (1) Apis.

Stridulous: (1) Gels.; (2) ign., mosch., samb.; *evening, on falling asleep:* (1) Phos.

Suffocative: (1) Ant-t., Hep., Lach., Meph., Phos., Spong., Samb.; (2) ars., chin., ip., merc-c., sil., sul.; *night:* (1) Ars., Samb., Lach., Phos.; (2) ant-t., dig., spong., sul.; *lying, while:* (1) Ars.; (2) graph.; *3 a. m.:* (1) Ant-t., Kali-c.; *emphysema in:* (1) Am-c.; *lying, while:* (1) Ars.; *measles, from suppressed:* (1) Cham.; *moving or raising the arms:* (2) spig.; *sleep, on falling:* (2) lach., spong.; *fears going to:* (2) grind., lach.; *swallowing, on:* (2) bell., cupr.

Superficial: (1) Phos.

Weak: (1) Mur-ac.; (2) camph., gels., phos., tuberc.

Wheezing: (1) Ip., Ars., Kali-c., Carb-v.; (2) brom., chin., dros., kali-a., nat-a., samb., syph.; *daytime:* (2) lyc.; *on lying down:* (2) ars.; *midnight, after:* (2) samb.; *during expiration:* (2) lyc.; *inspiring, while:* (2) chin., kali-c.

Whistling: (1) Chin.; (2) kali-c., samb., sang., spong., sul.; *morning*: (2) lach.; *inspiration*, *during*: (2) kali-c.; *whooping cough*, *in*: (2) cupr.

CHEST.

Abscess, AXILLA: (1) Merc., Hep., Sil.; (2) calc., nit-ac., sul. LUNGS: (1) Hep., Sil., Calc.; (2) kali-c., sul. MAMMÆ: (1) Phyt., Sil., Sul.; (2) bell., bry., lach., merc., phos.; *threatening in old cicatrices:* (1) Graph., Phyt.

Adhesion *of lungs after inflammation:* (2) ran-b.; *sensation of:* (2) kali-c., thuja.

Affections *of heart in general:* (1) Acon., Cact., Naja, Lach., Spig., Spong.; (2) aur., lith., lobel., puls.; *organic (see "Murmurs"):* (1) Cact., Naja, Kalm., Spig.; (2) lach., rhus-t., spong.

Alternating *with eye symptoms:* (1) Sil.

Aneurism *of the heart:* (1) Cact.

Angina pectoris: (1) Ars., Cact., Naja, Spig., Spong., Phos., Arn.; (2) am-c., apis, arg-n., aur., kalm., nux-v., ox-ac.

Anxiety *in:* (1) Acon., Ars., Phos.; *evening:* (1) Puls.; (2) phos.; *night:* (1) Puls., Ars.; *emotion agg.:* (1) Phos.; *lying on back, while:* (2) sul.; *on left side, while:* (1) Puls.; *playing piano, while:* (2) nat-c. HEART, *region of:* (1) Acon., Phos., Ant-t., Camph., Kalm.; (2) carb-v., ign., ip., spig., spong.; *2 a. m.:* (2) kali-c.; *evening:* (2) puls.; *night:* (1) Ars.; *moving about agg.:* (2) dig.; *sitting, while:* (2) caust.

Atrophy, *mammæ:* (1) Con., Kali-i.

Cancer, *mammæ:* (1) Con., Graph., Merc.; (2) apis, ars., aster., lach., phos., phyt., sil.

Catarrh: (1) Ars., Nux-v., Puls., Merc., Sang., Ant-t., Kali-bi.; (2) bry., dulc., hep., sul.

Clothing *agg.:* (1) Lach.

Coldness, *air, cold, breathing:* (2) cor-r.; *chill, during:* (2) caps.; *drinking, after:* (2) elaps; *expectoration, after:* (2) zinc.; *internal:* (2) ars.; *pain, at seat of:* (2) cact.

Congestion (*hyperæmia of chest*): (1) Acon., Bell., Ferr-ph., Cact., Phos., Spong., Sul.; (2) bry., dig., ip., lach., nux-v., sep., tereb.; *night:* (2) ferr., puls.; *alternating with congestion of the head:* (2) glon.; *climaxis, at:* (1) Lach.; *consumption, in:* (1) Ferr-ph.; *exertion, after:* (2) spong.; *lying down impossible:* (1) Cact., Bell.; *motion, after:* (2) spong.; *pregnancy, during:* (2) glon., nat-m., sep.; *uterine hemorrhage, after:* (2) aur-m., chin.; *waking, on:* (1) Lach. HEART, *rush of blood to:* (1) Glon.

Constriction, *tension, tightness:* (1) Acon., Ars., Cact., Lach., Sul., Phos., Bry.; (2) bell., brom., chel., graph., ign., lobel., lyc.; *evening:* (2) ars., puls., stann.; *in bed:* (2) ars.; *night:* (2) ferr., mez., puls.; *ascending:* (1) Ars.; *band, as from:* (1) Cact., Acon., Phos.; (2) amyl-n., ars., lobel.; *chill, during:* (1) Nux v.; (2) ars.; *convulsive:* (1) Asaf., Bell.; *cough, during:* (1) Phos.; (2) con., mag-ph., myrt., sul.; *cough, inclination to, from:* (2) sep.; *cough, spasmodic, during:* (2) mosch.; *drawing shoulders back amel.:* (2) calc.; *exertion,* *from:* (2) ars., nat-m.; *falling asleep, when:* (2) lach.; *manual labor, from:* (2) calc.; *masturbation, after:* (2) con.; *respiration, during:* (2) coc-c.; *spasmodic:* (1) Ign.; (2) cupr.; *anger, from:* (2) cupr.; *whooping cough in:* (2) caust., spong.; *swallowing:* (2) kali-c.; *talking, after:* (2) hep.; *talking, preventing:* (2) cact.; *waking, on:* (1) Lach.; (2) lact.; *walking, while:* (1) Ars.; (2) dig., kali-c.; *walking, rapid:* (2) puls.; *walking in open air amel.:* (2) puls. LOWER *part:* (1) Cact.; (2) dros., nux-v., spig. HEART: (1) Cact., Ars., Iod.; (2) spig., spong.; *drinking water amel.:* (2) phos.; *grasping sensation:* (1) Cact.; (2) iod., lil-t., nux-m., spig.; *as from a band of iron:* (2) cact.; *as from a hand:* (1) Cact., Iod.; (2) laur.; *or squeezed in a vise:* (1) Lil-t.; (2) spig., tarent.; *grief, after:* (2) ign.; *extending to back:* (2) lil-t.

Cyanosis: (1) Lach., Laur.; (2) ant-t., dig., ip.

Dilatation *of heart:* (1) Cact.; (2) apis, lach., naja, nat-m.

Discoloration, *yellow:* (2) chel. MAMMÆ, *blueness of ulcerated:* (2) lach.

Distension: (1) Bell., Lach.

Dropsy: (1) Ars., Apis, Bry., Merc-sul., Kal-c., Hell., Colch.; (2) aspar., dig., kali-i., lyc., merc., ran-b., seneg., squil., sul.; *side, can lie only on affected:* (2) ars. PERICARDIUM: (1) Ars., Dig., Colch.; (2) apis, apoc., sul.

Ebullition: (1) Amyl-n., Glon.; (2) acon., mill.

Emaciation, CLAVICLES: (1) Nat-m., Lyc. MAMMÆ: (2) con., iod.

Emphysema: (1) Ant-t., Ars., Hep., Lach., Lobel.; (2) dig., phos.

Emptiness, *sensation of:* (1) Stann.; (2) cocc., ign., sep.; *night:* (1) Sep.; *cough, during:* (2) sep., stann.; *expectoration, after:* (2) stann., zinc.; *sing, on beginning to:* (2) stann.

Empyema: (1) Ars., Merc., Sil.; (2) hep., kali-c., sul.

Eruptions: (1) Psor.; (2) ars., graph., nat-s., petr., sul.; *blood blisters:* (2) ars.; *boils:* (1) Kali-i.; *brown blotches:* (1) Sep.; (2) lyc., petr., phos.; *dry:* (1) Psor.; *herpes:* (2) graph., hep., petr., syph.; *zona:* (2) graph., lach., rhus-t., mez.; *rash:* (1) Led.; *red rash:* (1) Chel. AXILLA, *boils:* (1) Hep.; (2) merc., phos., sil.; *left:* (2) phos.; sep.; *recurrent:* (2) lyc.; *burning:* (2) merc.; *cracks:* (2) hep.; *dry:* (2) hep.; *scabs:* (1) Nat-m.

Expand, *lungs, desire to:* (1) Bry., Apis, Dig.

Fluttering: (1) Nat-m., Naja, Lil-t.; (2) lach., sul.; *ascending steps:* (1) Calc.; *lying, while:* (1) Nat-m.; *on left side:* (2) cact., dig., nat-m.; *waking, on:* (2) kali-i.

Fullness: (1) Acon., Apis, Lach., Sul.; (2) bry., ferr-ph., phos.; *morning:* (2) sul.; *evening:* (1) Puls.; (2) sul.; *in bed:* (2) nat-p.; *menses, before:* (1) Sul.

Gangrene *of lungs:* (1) Ars., Kreos.; (2) carbo-v., chin., lach., phos.

Heat, *flushes:* (2) glon., sep.; *rising up:* (2) sul.

Heaviness (*see "oppression"*): (1) Aur., Phos., Sul.

Inflammation *bronchial tubes (bronchitis):* (1) Acon., Bell., Bry., Ferr-ph., Phos., Ant t., Hep.; *aged people:* (2) am-c., camph., lyc. LUNGS: (1)

Acon., Bry., Phos., Verat-v., Ferr-ph., Sul., Ant-t.; (2) ars., carb-v., chel., hyos., lyc., merc., rhus-t.; *right:* (1) Bry.; (2) chel., kali-c., merc.; *lower lobe:* (2) kali-c., merc.; *left:* (2) lach., nat-s.; *left lower lobe:* (2) nat-s.; *abuse of aconite, after:* (2) bry.; *aged persons:* (2) bry., dig., hyos., nat-s., op., seneg.; *drunkards:* (2) hyos., nux-v., op.; *infants:* (1) Ip.; (2) acon., ant-t., bry., ferr-ph., merc., phos.; *neglected:* (1) Sul., Lyc., Sil.; (2) phos.; *nervous patients, in very:* (2) ant-t., bry., lyc., phos., rhus-t.; *pleuro-pneumonia:* (1) Bry., Phos., Ant-t.; (2) sul.; *sycotic-pneumonia:* (1) Nat-s.; *typhoid:* (1) Bry., Rhus-t., Hyos., Ant-t., Lyc., Phos., Sang.; *weakness, from loss of fluids:* (2) chin. PLEURA: (1) Acon., Bry., Sul.; (2) kali-c., merc., phos., squil.; *left:* (2) Kali-ind.; *old people*: (2) Nat-ac.; *Rheumatic*: (1) Bry., Ant-tart.: (2) Ars., sul.

Œdema, *pulmonary:* (1) Ant-t., Ars., Merc-sul., Lach.; (2) apis, dig., kali-i., phos.

Oppression: (1) Acon., Phos., Sul., Bry., Bell., Ars., Carb-v.; (2) apis, cact., chel., ferr., ip., puls., sep.; *bed, in:* (2) phos.; *waking, on:* (2) lach., nat-s.; *evening:* (1) Puls., Sep.; *bed, in:* (2) apis, *night:* (2) op., phos., rhus-t.; *walking in open air, after:* (2) phos.; *ascending:* (1) Acon., Ars., (2) calc.; *bending backward, amel.:* (1) Sul.; *changes, when weather, to cold:* (1) Ars.; *chill, during:* (1) Apis; *clothing agg.:* (1) Lach., Ars., Chel.; *coughing, when:* (1) Phos., Dros.; (2) ars., sul.; *inspiring, on:* (1) Spig., Phos.; *lying, while, head low, with:* (1) Spong.; *motion, on fast:* (1) Acon., Ars.; (2)

puls.; *throwing back shoulders, amel.:* (1) Calc.; *sleep, during:* (1) Lach.; *sleep, waking from:* (1) Kali-i.; (2) ars., nat-s.; *stormy weather:* (1) Ars.; *talking, while:* (1) Dros.; *walking, on:* (1) Ars.; *walking in open air, while:* (2) aur., phos.; *walking, after:* (1) Phos.; *walking quickly:* (1) Ars.; (2) puls.; *warm room:* (1) Apis.

Pain: (1) Bry., Phos., Bell., Spig., Spong.; (2) acon., cact., caust., kali-c., sang., sul.; *cough, during:* (1) Bry., Phos., Caust., Dros., Sul., Spong., Stann.; (2) acon., bell., bor., carb-v., kali-n., lyc., nat-s., sang., squil.; *fasting, from:* (2) iod.; *herpes zoster, after:* (2) mez., ran-b.; *inspiration, during:* (1) Acon., Bry., Bor., Squil.; (2) ars., phos.; *inspiration, agg.:* (1) Bry.; *lying, while, abdomen, on, amel.:* (2) bry.; *can lie only on back:* (2) acon., phos.; *lying on side amel.:* (1) Bry.; *lying on sound side:* (1) Puls.; *lying on left side:* (1) Phos., Spig.; *right side:* (1) Merc.; (2) bor.; *can lie only on right side:* (1) Spig.; (2) kali-c., naja; *motion agg.:* (1) Bry., Spig.; *pressure of hand amel.:* (1) Bry., Dros.; (2) eup-per., nat-s.; *respiration, on:* (1) Bry., Kali-c., Psor., Bor.; (2) lyc., spig., stann.; *deep:* (1) Bry., Kali-c., Nat-m.; (2) bor., caust., phos., sang.; *rising up in bed, on:* (1) Phos.; *rubbing amel.:* (2) phos.; *sitting:* (1) Seneg.; (2) bry.; *sneezing:* (2) bry., caust., dros.; *speaking:* (1) Bor.; *splinter, as if:* (1) Arg-n.; *turning:* (1) Ran-b.; *weather changing:* (1) Ran-b. SIDES, *right:* (1) Chel.; (2) calc., sang.; *apex of right lung:* (1) Ars.; *left:* (1) Phos., Ran-b.; (2) cact., cimic., lach., nat-s.; *4 p. m.:* (1)

Lyc.; *cough, during:* (1) Bry., Merc.; (2) arn., phos., puls.; *inspiration:* (1) Bry., Squil.; (2) chel., kali-c.; *laughing:* (1) Bry.; *lying down, when:* (2) puls.; *lying down on back amel.:* (2) phos.; *lying on left side:* (1) Phos.; *motion, on:* (1) Bry.; (2) ran-b.; *pressure amel.:* (2) bry., phos.; *respiration:* (1) Bry.; *deep:* (1) Kal-c.; (2) acon., bry.; *speaking:* (1) Bor.; *walking:* (1) Ran-b. LOWER: (1) Puls.; (2) rhus-t.; *right:* (2) chel., merc-c.; *left:* (2) cact., kali-ph. LUNGS: (2) lyc., sul., tuberc.; *as if lobe were adhering to ribs:* (2) kali-c.; *left:* (2) sul.; *evening agg.:* (2) sul.; *above nipple:* (1) Sul., Arum-t.; *apex, right:* (1) Ars. STERNUM: (2) bell., bry., sul.; *coughing, when:* (1) Bry.; (2) phos., sang., sul.; *behind:* (1) Sang.; (2) eup-per.; *extending to back:* (1) Kali-bi. HEART, *aching:* (2) arn., bell., phos. BRUISED: (1) Arn., Bry., Calc., Puls., Ran-b.; (2) apis; *morning:* (2) staph.; *moving, on:* (2) staph.; *coughing, on:* (1) Bry., Arn.; (2) phos.; *respiration, during:* (1) Arn.; *touch agg.:* (1) Arn., Ran-b. BURNING: (1) Ars., Phos., Sul.; (2) apis, canth., carb-v.; *coals, as from glowing:* (1) Carb-v.; (2) lach.; *coughing, during:* (1) Spong., Iod.; *dry cough:* (1) Iod., Spong.; *rising flushes face:* (1) Sul.; *extending to face:* (1) Sul.; *extending upward:* (1) Sul. SIDES, *right:* (1) Bry.; (2) bell.; *left:* (1) Phos., Ran-b.; *lying on left side agg.:* (2) phos. CUTTING (*sharp pains*): (1) Kali-c.; *evening:* (1) Kali-c.; *evening, after lying down:* (1) Kali-c.; *coughing:* (2) bry., nat-m., sul.; *eating, after:*

(2) nux-v.; *lying on right side agg.:* (2) kali-c.; *lying on left side agg.:* (2) phos. PRESSING: (1) Sul.; (2) phos.; *inspiration, deep, on:* (1) Kali-c., Spong. RAWNESS (*includes trachea and bronchia*): (1) Caust., Phos., Nux-v.; (2) sul.; *coughing, when:* (2) caust., carb-v., phos., rumex. RHEUMATIC: (1) Bry., Rhus-t., Ran-b, Spig.; (2) cimic., colch., rumex. SORENESS: (1) Arn., Caust., Bry., Ran-b.; (2) eup-per., phos., rhus-t., sul.; *evening, menses before and during:* (1) Zinc.; *cough, during:* (1) Arn., Bry.; (2) calc., eup-per., nat-s., phos.; *coughing, from:* (1) Arn., Carb-v., Phos., Spong., Stann.; (2) bry., caust., dros., eup-per., nat-s., sul.; *holds chest with hands during cough:* (1) Arn., Bry.; (2) nat-s.; *inspiring:* (1) Bry., Calc.; (2) eup-per.; *lying agg.:* (1) Chin.; *menses, before and during:* (1) Zinc.; *percussion agg.:* (1) Chin.; *pressing amel.:* (2) bry., dros., eup per., nat-m., nat-s.; *respiration:* (2) calc., kali-c.; *sitting upright and holding chest amel.:* (1) Bry.; (2) nat-s.; *touch:* (1) Calc., Chin., Ran-b.; (2) kali-c.; *turning in the bed, on:* (1) Ran-b.; *after a restless night:* (2) bry. STITCHING: (1) Acon., Bry., Kali-c., Squil., Spig., Sul., Phos.; (2) merc., nat-m., ran-b.; *coughing:* (1) Bry., Merc., Squil., Bor.; (2) acon., bell., dros., iod., sul.; *fever, during:* (1) Bry.; (2) kali-c.; *inspiring:* (1) Acon., Bry., Bor., Squil.; (2) kali-c., phos.; *can lie only on the back:* (2) acon., bry., phos.; *lying, side, right, on the, amel.:* (1) Spig.; *lying, side, left, on the:* (1) Phos., Spig.; *motion, during:* (1) Bry., Spig.; *pressure with*

the hand amel.: (1) Bry., Dros.; *respiration, on:* (1) Bry., Bor., Kali-c.; (2) spig., squil.; *respiration, on deep:* (1) Bry., Nat-m., Kali-c.; (2) acon., bor., kali-n., phos., sul.; *rest agg.:* (1) Rhus-t.; *rest amel.:* (1) Bry.; *rubbing amel.:* (2) phos.; *sneezing agg.:* (1) Merc.; (2) dros.; *touch:* (1) Ran-b.; *turning, by:* (1) Ran-b.; *weather, changing, agg.:* (1) Ran-b.; *extending to back:* (1) Sul. ANTERIOR, *part, coughing, on:* (1) Merc. SIDES: (1) Bry., Kali-c., Squil.; (2) acon., phos., sul.; *right:* (1) Bry., Bor., Chel.; (2) kali-c., sul.; *right side amel.:* (1) Phos.; *lower part:* (2) kali-c.; *lying on the back:* (2) sul.; *lying on the right side, when:* (2) acon.; *respiration, during:* (1) Bry., Bor.; *left side:* (1) Phos., Sul., Rumex, Stann.; *lying on left side agg.:* (2) phos. stann.; *morning:* (2) bry.; *walking rapidly agg.:* (2) sul.; *afternoon, motion, on:* (1) Bry.; *night:* (1) Con., Lyc.; (2) sul., puls.; *ascending steps:* (2) staph.; *asthma, during:* (2) arn.; *coughing:* (1) Bry., Merc.; (2) arn., kali-c., sul.; *inspiration:* (1) Bry., Kali-c., Squil.; (2) acon., bor., spig., sul.; *lying, when:* (2) puls.; *lying left side agg.:* (2) stann.; *motion, during:* (1) Bry.; *respiration, deep:* (2) acon., bry., kali-c., sul.; *speaking, after:* (1) Bor.; *standing, while:* (2) nat-s.; *walking:* (1) Ran-b.; *extending, scapula, to:* (1) Sul.; *shoulders, to:* (2) kali-c., sang. STERNUM: (1) Ars.; (2) bry., kali-i., sul.; *coughing, on:* (1) Bry.; (2) psor.; *deep breathing:* (1) Caust.; (2) bry., nat-m.; *sitting, bent, while:* (2) rhus-t.

Paralysis, LUNGS: (1) Ant-t., Carb-v., Bar-c., Lach., Lyc.; *old people:* (1) Bar-c., Chin.; (2) phos.

Perspiration: (1) Calc., Bov., Kali-n., Selen.; (2) phos-ac., phos.

Phthisis: (1) Sul., Calc., Lyc., Psor., Tuberc., Calc-ph., Stann., Sil., Kali-c., Hep.; (2) iod., myrt., phos-ac., sang., sep., spong., ther., zinc.; *acute:* (1) Ferr-ph., Puls., Sil.; (2) bry., phos., sul.; *menses, suppressed, from:* (1) Senec.; *emaciation:* (1) Iod.; *florida:* (2) ferr., puls., ther.; *hæmorrhages, after:* (2) chin.; *incipient:* (1) Sul., Puls., Tuberc., Phos., Hep., Lyc., Sil., Kali-c., Psor.; (2) bry., senec.; *last stage:* (1) Lyc., Carb-v., Sang., Calc., Puls., Tarent.; (2) chin., lach., phos., pyrog.; *nursing mothers:* (2) kali-c.; *old people:* (2) nat-s.; *pituitous:* (2) ant-c., ant-t., euon., ferr-ph., hep., kali-i., kali-chl., lyc., phos., psor., sang., senec., stann.; *purulent and ulcerative:* (1) Calc., Lyc., Phos.; (2) hep., kali-c., puls., sil., sul.; *sycotic:* (1) Thuja, Nat-s., Nit-ac., Calc., Lyc.; *tuberculous deposits to delay*: (2) calc., kali-c., lyc., phos., puls., stann.

Shocks, *cough, with:* (1) Lyc.

Spots, *liver:* (1) Lyc.; *mottled:* (1) Lach., Crot-h.

Suppuration *of lungs:* (1) Sil., Hep., Calc., Phos.; (2) kali-c., lyc., psor., tuberc.; *acute:* (2) psor., puls.

Weakness: (1) Stann., Carb-v.; (2) kali-c., phos-ac., phos., sul.; *morning on waking:* (1) Carb-v.; *cough, from:* (1) Stann.; (2) nit-ac., phos-ac., psor.; *exertion, after:* (1) Spong.; *expectoration, after:* (1) Stann.; *sing, on beginning to:* (1) Stann.; *speaking, after:* (1) Stann.; (2) sul.; *waking, on:* (1) Carb-v.

INDEX.